Sports Skill Analysis

Guided by the conceptualization of content knowledge, this book covers sports analysis (identification of techniques and tactics), skill analysis (identification of critical elements, observation, evaluation of students' performance through error detection, and interventions), and biomechanical principles and their applications to skill performance and analysis, which teachers or coaches need to possess for effective teaching and coaching.

The importance for preservice and in-service physical education teachers or coaches to acquire in-depth content knowledge is supported by national standards and research. Studies have shown that an improvement in preservice and in-service physical education teachers' specialized content knowledge leads to an increase in their pedagogical content knowledge, which results in better learning and performance among students. Practical examples for conducting sports and skill analysis, designing teaching progressions for interventions, and applying biomechanical principles are provided.

This book equips teachers or coaches with knowledge and skills to conduct sports and skill analysis, which are essential for effective teaching and coaching, and will be key reading for undergraduate and graduate students majoring in physical education teacher education and sports coaching and in-service physical education teachers and current coaches.

Weidong Li is a Professor at the Department of Human Sciences at the Ohio State University, USA. Dr. Li is a research fellow of AAHPERD (currently renamed as the Society of Health and Physical Educator) and Physical Activity and Public Health Research Course sponsored by the Centers for Disease Control and Prevention. In 2020, Dr. Li was awarded SHAPE North America Society Fellow. From 2014 to 2018, Dr. Li served as an editor of the *Journal of Teaching in Physical Education*.

Boyi Dai is a Professor in the Division of Kinesiology and Health at the University of Wyoming, USA. Dr. Dai's research is focused on jump-landing biomechanics and anterior cruciate ligament injuries, exoskeleton and low-back loading, and tripping and falls. Dr. Dai is a fellow of and serves as a Vice President (Research and Projects) for the International Society of

Biomechanics in Sports. He also serves as an Associate Editor for *Sports Biomechanics*.

Qin Zhu is a Professor in the Division of Kinesiology and Health at the University of Wyoming, USA. Using a perception-action approach, Dr. Zhu's research addresses learning and control mechanisms underlying the functional movements often seen in daily life or sport settings. He served as an advisory board member for the *Journal of Sports Sciences* and the external grant reviewer for NIH and NSF. When he is not wearing an academic hat, he is a certified high-performance coach by USA Badminton and a certified umpire by Badminton Pan American Confederation.

Sports Skill Analysis

Weidong Li, Boyi Dai, and Qin Zhu

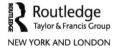
Routledge
Taylor & Francis Group

NEW YORK AND LONDON

First published 2024
by Routledge
605 Third Avenue, New York, NY 10158

and by Routledge
4 Park Square, Milton Park, Abingdon, Oxon, OX14 4RN

Routledge is an imprint of the Taylor & Francis Group, an informa business

ISBN: 978-1-032-36439-1 (hbk)
ISBN: 978-1-032-36436-0 (pbk)
ISBN: 978-1-003-33196-4 (ebk)

DOI: 10.4324/9781003331964

Typeset in Times New Roman
by MPS Limited, Dehradun

Contents

Figures

Tables

Preface

Teachers or coaches must know their content to effectively teach or coach sports. However, evidence shows that teachers in physical education or coaches lack content knowledge. Developing content knowledge among physical education teachers or coaches is one of the most challenging tasks for teacher education (Siedentop, 2002) or sports coaching programs. The importance for physical education teachers or coaches to acquire in-depth content knowledge is reflected in national standards for physical education teacher education and sports coaching and is supported by research.

According to Ward (2009), content knowledge for sports can be sorted into four domains: (a) knowledge of rules and etiquette (i.e., knowing the rules for double dribbling in basketball), (b) knowledge of techniques and tactics (i.e., knowing the critical elements of dribbling and shooting techniques and fast break in basketball), (c) knowledge of student errors (i.e., knowing the common mistakes made by students and common approaches to fix them), (d) knowledge of instructional tasks and representations (i.e., task instructions and demonstrations, and teaching progressions used to teach a skill). In general, an individual needs to know Domains of (a) and (b) to play sports. To teach or coach sports, an individual must be trained in Domains (c) and (d) to acquire the specific specialized content knowledge.

Using the conceptualization of content knowledge (Shulman, 1989; Ball, Thames, & Phelps, 2008; Ward, 2009), this book intends to develop in-depth content knowledge among physical education teachers and coaches by focusing on sports skill analysis, which are essential for effective teaching or coaching. Teachers or coaches must know what are techniques and tactics to teach or coach, identify critical elements of a specific skill, observe and record performance, evaluate and diagnose performance by identifying the common errors and its causes and the strength areas, understand the biomechanical principles underlying the common errors, understand how students or athletes learn motor skills, and then use these principles and motor learning theories to develop interventions and tasks progressions to correct these errors.

This book consists of four sections with 16 chapters. Section 1 has two chapters. Chapter 1 introduces the conceptual framework for sports and skill analysis, describes the definitions of sport analysis and skill analysis, and discusses the importance of content knowledge and pedagogical content knowledge. Chapter 2 discusses different approaches to skill analysis and introduces models of qualitative skill analysis. Section 2 has six chapters, which focuses on the first component of integrative biomechanical model of qualitative skill analysis preparation. Chapter 3 introduces the definition of preparation and discusses five major knowledge bases for the teacher or coach to possess, including knowledge of performers, knowledge of sports skill, knowledge of the biomechanical model of the skill, knowledge of effective instructions, and knowledge of motor learning and control. Chapter 4 defines sports analysis, skill, technique, and tactics, discusses the similarities and differences among skills, techniques, and tactics, and introduces steps to successfully conduct sports analysis. Chapter 5 focuses on understanding the movement preparation, specifically, a cognitive process that precedes the production of a skillful movement and introduces the theoretical models and behavioural measures of movement preparation, as well as the factors that influence movement preparation. Chapter 6 focuses on understanding the control mechanism underlying skilled movements and two motor control mechanisms are introduced. Chapter 7 focuses on understanding motor learning from the learner's perspective. Two models of stages of learning will be introduced. Different kinds of performance measures are discussed to help with detecting motor learning. Chapter 8 defines what is task progressions, introduces the concept of task and task development, discusses factors that affect task complexity and how to design teaching progressions. Section 3 covers biomechanical concepts and principles and their applications to skill analysis with five chapters. Chapter 9 describes basic biomechanical concepts. Chapter 10 focuses on biomechanical principles in linear kinematics and their applications to skill analysis. Chapter 11 focuses on biomechanical principles in angular kinematics and their applications to skill analysis. Chapter 12 focuses on biomechanical principles in linear kinetics and their applications to skill analysis. Chapter 13 focuses on biomechanical principles in angular kinetics and their applications to skill analysis. Section 4 covers the final three components of integrative biomechanical model of qualitative skill analysis: observation, evaluation and diagnosis, and intervention. Chapter 14 defines observation and discusses effective strategies for observation and steps to conduct effective observations. Chapter 15 defines evaluation and diagnosis and discusses how to conduct evaluation and diagnosis based on biomechanical principles and prioritize errors for interventions. Chapter 16 presents the last component of intervention and discusses a variety of intervention methods to correct errors for better performance.

The conceptualization of this book is based on the first author's 15-year teaching of this Skill Analysis course to undergraduate and graduate students in Physical Education Teacher Education and Sports Coaching programs and research on content knowledge in physical education. This book is conceptually based by adopting content knowledge and pedagogical content knowledge as the conceptual framework. It is comprehensive by providing a broad knowledge bases for teachers or coaches to successfully conduct skill analysis for better performance. It is also practical by providing examples help teachers or coaches better understand theories, principles, and concepts and how to apply them to conduct sports and skill analysis for better performance.

Acknowledgments

I devote this book to my parents, son, daughter, and brother for their love and support throughout my life journey. I want to thank my coauthors, Dr. Boyi Dai and Dr. Qin Zhu, who have been working with me on this book for the past two years. It has been a long journey, but also a fun and exciting one.

Section 1

Sports and skill analysis

Conceptual framework and definitions

This section focuses on the conceptual framework and definitions of sports and skill analysis, which has two chapters. Chapter 1 introduces the conceptual framework for sports and skill analysis, describes the definitions of sport analysis and skill analysis, and discusses the importance of content knowledge and pedagogical content knowledge. Chapter 2 discusses different approaches to skill analysis and introduces models of qualitative skill analysis.

DOI: 10.4324/9781003331964-1

1 Conceptual framework for sports and skill analysis

Content knowledge

Outcomes

- Understand the definitions and classifications of content knowledge.
- Understand what pedagogical content knowledge is.
- Understand the relationship between content knowledge and pedagogical content knowledge.
- Recognize the importance of developing competence in sports and skill analysis among pre-service physical education teachers or coaches.

Definitions of sports and skill analysis

To teach or coach sports effectively, teachers or coaches must know the content and can adapt the instruction to the needs of their students or athletes. In this book, we introduce two critical skills that teachers or coaches must have for effective teaching or coaching. They are sports analysis and skill analysis. Sports analysis is the process of systematically identifying, analyzing, and sequencing all the components in a sport necessary for effective teaching or coaching. It consists of five domains: (1) physiological training and conditioning, (2) background knowledge, (3) psychomotor skills (techniques and tactics), (4) progressive practices, and (5) psycho-social concepts. We will discuss sports analysis in Chapter 4 in detail.

A core teaching or coaching practice for effective teaching or coaching is to make instructional adaptations to the needs of students or athletes. To adapt the instruction to the needs of students or athletes in motor skill performance, teachers or coaches must possess the ability to prepare, observe, evaluate, and diagnose skill performances by identifying correct and incorrect performance responses, and design interventions to improve students' or athletes' skill performance based on the biomechanical model of the skills. This is called skill analysis. Skill analysis is a complicated process. More detailed information about skill analysis is presented later in Chapter 2.

DOI: 10.4324/9781003331964-2

Importance of sports and skill analysis

Why do teachers or coaches need the skills to conduct sports and skill analysis? First, let us look at why a teacher or coach needs to learn how to conduct sports analysis. The main rationale is for effective teaching or coaching. To effectively teach or coach a sport, physical education teachers or coaches must know the content. Through sports analysis, we produce a knowledge package. This knowledge package consists of common content knowledge and specialized content knowledge related to a sport that a teacher or coach needs to effectively teach or coach to students or athletes. The importance of possessing content knowledge for teachers or coaches for effective teaching or coaching will be discussed after introducing the theoretical framework of content knowledge and pedagogical content knowledge later in this chapter.

The importance of developing skill analysis competency is highlighted in research on coaching education and methods. A review by Griffo et al. (2019) showed that 47.5% of studies focused on the topic of coaching education and methods. The operational definition of coaching education is "Research that encompasses the methods in which coaches utilize in their fields when designing scaffolded practices and game plans (e.g., exercises, strategies, plays). Developing skills and knowledge, differences in roles between coaches and educators (specifically physical educators)" (p. 108). The operational definition of coach education is "Research that aims to increase coaches' understanding and learning of their sport (e.g., suggestions and empirical-based information for coaches). Additionally, assessing and enhancing the effectiveness of coaching education programs. Last, research that includes the impact that coach education has on teams and players" (p. 108). Many of those competencies identified in those studies are related to sports and skill analysis. In another study by McCleery et al. (2022), the findings from the Delphi panel of expert coaches identified 15 ambitious coaching core practices for effective coaching. Among those core practices, diagnosis, feedback, adapting instruction, and sequence are all part of skill analysis competency.

Physical education literature has clearly identified the reasons why teachers need to develop skill analysis competency. As pointed out in the article by Ward et al. (2021), there are four main reasons. The first one comes from research evidence. Studies have shown that preservice physical education teachers often lack skill analysis competency to detect errors by discriminating between actual and desired performance (Hoffman, 1987; Lounsbery & Coker,2008; Wilkinson, 1992; Williams & Rink, 2003). This impedes teachers' ability to make instructional adaptations to the needs of individual students, thus restraining student learning and performance (Ward et al., 2021).

The second reason for teachers to develop skill analysis competence is related to teaching outcomes of school physical education (Ward et al., 2021). The SHAPE of America K–12 physical education standards state, "The physically literate individual demonstrates competency in a variety of motor skills and movement patterns" (SHAPE America – Society of Health and Physical Educators, 2017). Developing students' motor skill competence is one of the important outcomes of school physical education. Students with higher levels of motor skill competence are more likely to participate in physical activity (De Meester et al., 2016; Lounsbery & Coker, 2008). To develop students' motor skill competence, physical education teachers should possess competence in sports and skill analyses, thus being able to develop content, detect errors, and provide interventions to fix errors for better skill competence.

Thirdly, physical education teachers need skill analysis competency to conduct student learning assessments (Ward et al., 2021). Assessments can be done at the end of the unit or semester which is called summative assessments. For assessments that are done during the instructional unit, they are called formative assessments. Competency in skill analysis enables physical education teachers to conduct those formative and summative assessments, especially formative assessments. Physical education teachers provide constant feedback on students' skill performance to either reinforce what students perform correctly or correct their performance errors. Without competence in skill analysis, they will not be able to identify good performance components for reinforcement and errors for interventions to improve students' skill performance and learning. Physical education teachers often lack the requisite assessment knowledge and have trouble in conducting assessments (Matanin & Tannehill, 1994; Williams & Rink, 2003). Therefore, there is an urgent need to train in-service and pre-service teachers on how to conduct assessments. Skill analysis is an essential tool for teachers to use to conduct assessments.

Finally, the importance of developing teachers' competence in sports and skill analysis is also demonstrated in the National Standards for Initial Physical Education Teacher Education (SHAPE America, 2017; Ward et al., 2021). Standards 1, 4, and 5 state, "Physical education candidates demonstrate an understanding of common and specialized content and scientific and theoretical foundations for the delivery of an effective pre-K–12 physical education program", "Physical education candidates engage students in meaningful learning experiences through effective use of pedagogical skills. They use communication, feedback, and instructional and managerial skills to enhance student learning", and "Physical education candidates select and implement appropriate assessments to monitor students' progress and guide decision making related to instruction and learning" (SHAPE America, 2017).

Conceptual framework for sports and skill analysis: Content knowledge

Effective teaching or coaching promotes personal growth among students or athletes and maximizes their learning and sports performance. It also impacts students' or athletes' physical, social emotional, and behavioral well-being. Effective teaching or coaching is a complex work, which is influenced by numerous factors. Those factors include teaching or coaching experiences, educational levels, personalities, in-depth content knowledge and PCK, teaching or coaching philosophies, and available resources such as equipment and facilities, etc. Among those factors, content knowledge and PCK are two of the most critical factors that determine the effectiveness of teaching or coaching.

The concept of PCK originates from general education, which was first introduced by Shulman (1986) as an important concept to understand teaching effectiveness. Over the past 30 years, scholars in general education have proposed various conceptualizations of PCK. For example, Shulman (1987) conceptualizes PCK as a blending of content and pedagogy, which teachers can utilize to adapt and present content and knowledge to learners with diverse interests and abilities. Grossman (1990) conceptualized PCK as an amalgam of four teacher knowledge bases: (a) knowledge and beliefs about the purposes for teaching; (b) knowledge of students, including students' characteristics, cognitive abilities, perceptions, motivation; (c) knowledge of curricular and curriculum resources; and (d) knowledge of instructional strategies and representations for teaching a particular topic. Ball et al. (2008) conceptualized PCK as knowledge of the relationships among content, students, teaching, and curriculum, including (a) knowledge of content and students, (b) knowledge of content and teaching, and (c) knowledge of content and curriculum. The conceptualization of PCK has shifted its focus from a distinctive category of teacher knowledge base (Shulman, 1987) to an amalgam of teacher knowledge bases (Grossman, 1990; Ball et al., 2008).

In the coaching literature, Cassidy et al. (2016) discussed the importance of coaches acquiring PCK and content knowledge for effective coaching. The authors introduced the framework of PCK and content knowledge by Shulman (1986) in education and the work by Metzler (2000) in physical education to sports coaching. However, little research has been conducted in this area under the framework of PCK and CK.

PCK has been adapted and studied by scholars in physical education. In physical education, Ward et al. (2015) defined PCK as "a focal point, a locus, defined as such as an event in time (and therefore specific contextually) where teachers make decisions in terms of content based on their understandings of a number of knowledge bases (e.g., pedagogy, learning, motor development, students, contexts, and curriculum)" (p. 131). It is informed by a variety of knowledge bases, including knowledge of students, knowledge of curriculum, knowledge of content, knowledge of context, etc. PCK is situational and relational. That is, in a specific teaching moment, physical education teacher takes actions to improve students' learning and performance through decision-making based on analyzing the changing relationships among students, learning tasks, and environments. For example, a third-grade student just learns how to trap and pass a soccer ball to his or her partner and struggles to complete this task during practice. Physical education teacher decides to have him or her revisit trapping the ball since this student seems to have trouble in trapping the ball first. After this student shows some consistency in successfully trapping the ball, physical education teacher then has him or her practice the original trapping and passing learning task.

PCK is strongly influenced by levels of content knowledge. In general education, Ball et al. (2008) conceptualized content knowledge as subject matter knowledge, which consists of three domains: common content knowledge (CCK), specialized content knowledge (SCK), and horizon content knowledge (HCK). CCK refers to skills and knowledge that are needed to perform a task or an activity. For example, in mathematics, it is the ability to correctly solve problems such as 1+1=2. SCK refers to skills and knowledge that are needed to teach a task or an activity (Ball et al., 2008). For example, in mathematics, it is the ability to teach how to solve problems. That is, teaching students how to add 1+1=2. SCK includes skills and knowledge of how to represent mathematical reasoning and conduct error analysis and how to select, sequence, and implement instructional tasks. HCK refers to an understanding of the progressive relations among topics/tasks in the curriculum. For example, in mathematics, how are the learning tasks taught in grade 1 related to those taught in grade 2?

In physical education, Ward (2009) classified content knowledge for sports and physical activities into two main domains: CCK and SCK. CCK consists of knowledge of rules and etiquette (i.e., knowing the rules for double dribbling in basketball) and knowledge of techniques and tactics (i.e., knowing the critical elements of dribbling and shooting techniques and fast break in basketball). SCK consists of error detection (i.e., knowing the common mistakes made by students and common approaches to fix them under the guidance of biomechanical principles) and tasks and representations (i.e., task instructions and demonstrations, and task progressions used to teach a skill). In general, an individual needs to know CCK to perform an activity or a sport. To teach or coach a sport, an individual shall possess CCK and must be trained to acquire specific SCK.

Importance of content knowledge

Teachers or coaches must know content knowledge to effectively teach or coach sports. In the coaching literature, Cassidy et al. (2016) discussed the importance of coaches acquiring content knowledge for effective coaching. The authors introduced the framework of content knowledge by Shulman (1986) in education and the work by Metzler (2000) in physical education to sports coaching. Even though the National Standards for Sports Coaching does not specifically use the terms of content knowledge in the statement, it still emphasizes the importance for coaches to possess sport-specific knowledge. For example, the National standards for Sports Coaching states that sport coaches need to "draw upon current coaching science, sport-specific knowledge, and best practices to conduct quality sport practices, prepare athletes for competition, and effectively manage contests. This practice can be framed around how coaches plan, teach, assess, and adapt in practices and competition" (Gano-Overway et al., 2021, p10).

CK is placed at the center of teacher education as it is what teachers need to know to be able to teach physical education, and it lays a foundation for improving pedagogical content knowledge (Grossman et al., 2005: Shulman, 1986, Siedentop, 2002; Ward, 2009). The importance of content knowledge is highlighted in the NASPE/NCATE Standards for Initial Preparation of Physical Education Teachers (SHAPE of America, 2017). The standards require that "Physical education candidates demonstrate an understanding of common and specialized content, and scientific and theoretical foundations for the delivery of an effective preK–12 physical education program", and "Physical education candidates apply content and foundational knowledge to plan and implement developmentally appropriate learning experiences aligned with local, state and/or SHAPE America's National Standards and Grade-Level Outcomes for K–12 Physical Education through the effective use of resources, accommodations and/or modifications, technology and metacognitive strategies to address the diverse needs of all students."

The importance for preservice and in-service physical education teachers to acquire in-depth content knowledge is also supported by research evidence. There is strong evidence to support that an improvement in preservice and in-service physical education teachers' content knowledge leads to an increase in their PCK such as using more correct task representations and more mature tasks with more diverse forms of visual and verbal representations in teaching. Correspondingly, increased content knowledge and PCK in physical education teachers produce better learning and performance among students, including an improved throwing performance (Chang et al., 2020), an improved game performance in volleyball (Kim, 2016), increased correct skill trials in volleyball (Kim & Ko, 2020), and higher percentages of correct practice trials and lower percentages of incorrect practice trials in badminton (Iserbyt et al., 2017; Sinelnikov et al., 2016; Ward et al., 2015). Therefore, physical education teachers who possess in-depth content knowledge can improve their ability to design progressive instructional tasks, better represent instructions to students, provide appropriate feedback aligned with students' performance, and design interventions to correct students' errors in their skill performance, thus supporting and improve their students' understanding and application of skills in sports and game.

CK provides a conceptual framework for sports and skill analysis, where preservice physical education teachers or coaches are trained to develop expertise in CCK and SCK for effective teaching or coaching. Game rules and knowledge of technique and tactics play a significant role in laying a knowledge foundation for teachers or coaches to conduct sports and skill analysis. Teachers must know game rules, techniques, and tactics so that they can judge whether students or athletes perform them effectively and efficiently and then determine what is the next step of instruction. SCK contributes to skill analysis because it supports teachers or coaches in judging what to look for in students' performance, what appropriate tasks to select, how to sequence those learning tasks, how to present those learning tasks to students or athletes, and what interventions to develop to correct students' performance errors, thus improving students' learning and sports performance (Ward et al., 2021). This same principle also applies to coaches for effective coaching.

Summary

In this chapter, we discuss the definitions of content knowledge and PCK and their components. Content knowledge provides a conceptual framework for sports and skill analysis, consisting of CCK and SCK. The terms CCK and SCK are defined. The importance of teachers' possession of in-depth content knowledge is supported by national standards and strong research evidence. More research evidence to support the importance of developing coaches' content knowledge is needed.

Questions for reflection

- What is pedagogical content knowledge?
- What is content knowledge?
- What is the relationship between content knowledge and pedagogical content knowledge?
- What are the definitions of common content knowledge and specialized content knowledge? Please provide some examples for each term.
- Why is content knowledge important for physical education teachers coaches to possess?

References

Ball, D. L., Thames, M. H., & Phelps, G. (2008). Content knowledge for teaching: What makes it special? *Journal of Teacher Education*, *59*(5), 389–407.

Cassidy, T., Jones, R. L., & Potrac, P. *Understanding sports coaching: The Pedagogical, social, and cultural foundations of coaching practice* (3rd ed.). New York, NY: Taylor and Francis Group.

Chang, S. H., Ward, P., & Goodway, J. D. (2020). The effect of a content knowledge teacher professional workshop on enacted pedagogical content knowledge and student learning in a throwing unit. *Physical Education and Sport Pedagogy*, *25*(5), 493–508.

De Meester, A., Stodden, D., Brian, A., True, L., Cardon, G., Tallir, I., & Haerens, L. (2016). Associations among elementary school children's actual motor competence, perceived motor competence, physical activity, and BMI: A cross-sectional study. *PLoS One*, 1(10). 10.1371/journal.pone.0164600.

Gano-Overway, L., Thompson, M., & Van Mullem, P. (2021). *National Standards for sports coaches: Quality coaches, quality sports.* Annapolis Junction, MD: SHAPE of America.

Griffo, J. M., Jensen, M., Anthony, C. C., Baghurst, T., & Kulinna, P. H. (2019). A decade of research literature in sport coaching (2005–2015). *International Journal of Sports Science and Coaching, 14*(2), 205–215.

Grossman, P. L. (1990). *The making of a teacher: Teacher knowledge and teacher education*. New York: Teachers College Press.

Grossman, P., Schoenfeld, A., & Lee, C. (2005). Teaching subject matter: In L. Darling-Hammond, J. Bransford, P. LePage, K. Hammerness, & H. Duffy (Eds.), *Preparing teachers for a changing world: What teachers should learn and be able to do* (pp. 201–231). San Francisco: Jossey Bass.

Hoffman, S. (1987). Dreaming the impossible dream: The decline and fall of physical education. In J. D. Massengale (Ed.), *Trends toward the future in physical education* (pp. 121–135). Champaign, IL: Human Kinetics.

Iserbyt, P., Ward, P., & Li, W. (2017). Effects of improved content knowledge on pedagogical content knowledge and student performance in physical education. *Physical Education & Sport Pedagogy, 22*(1), 71–88.

Kim, I. (2016). Exploring changes to a teacher's teaching practices and student learning through a volleyball content knowledge workshop. *European Physical Education Review, 22*(2), 225–242.

Kim, I, & Ko, B. (2020). Content knowledge, enacted pedagogical content knowledge, and student performance between teachers with different levels of content expertise. *Journal of Teaching in Physical Education, 39*(1), 111–120.

Lounsbery, M., & Coker, C. (2008). Developing skill-analysis competency in physical education teachers. *Quest, 60*(2), 255–267.

Matanin, M., & Tannehill, D. (1994). Assessment and grading in physical education. *Journal of Teaching in Physical Education, 13*(4), 395–405.

McCleery, J., Hoffman, J. L., Tereschenko, I., & Pauketat, R. (2022). Ambitious coaching core practices: Borrowing from teacher education to inform coach development pedagogy. *International Sport Coaching Journal, 9*, 62–73.

Metzler, M. (2000). *Instructional models for physical education*. Needham Heights, MA: Allyn & Bacon.

SHAPE of America – Society of Health and Physical Educators. (2017). *National standards for initial physical education teacher education*. Retrieved from http://www.shapeamerica.org/accreditation/upload/National-Standards-for-Initial-Physical-Education-Teacher-Education-2017.pdf.

Shulman, L. (1986). Those who understand: Knowledge growth in teaching. *Educational Researcher, 15*(2), 4–14.

Shulman, L. (1987). Knowledge and teaching: Foundations of the reform. *Harvard Educational Review, 57*(1), 1–23.

Siedentop, D. (2002). Content knowledge for physical education. *Journal of Teaching in Physical Education, 21*, 368–377.

Sinelnikov, O. A., Kim, I., Ward, P., et al. (2016). Changing beginning teachers' content knowledge and its effects on student learning. *Physical Education & Sport Pedagogy, 21*(4), 425–440.

Ward, P. (2009). Content matters: Knowledge that alters teaching. In L. Housner, M. Metzler, P. Schempp, and T. Templin (Eds.), *Historic traditions and future directions of research on teaching and teacher education in physical education* (pp. 345–356). Morgantown, WV: Fitness Information Technology.

Ward, P., Ayvazo, S., Dervent, F., Iserbyt, P., Kim, I., & Li, W. (2021). Skill analysis for teachers: Considerations for physical education teacher education. *Journal of Physical Education, Recreation & Dance, 92*(2), 15–21.

Ward, P., Kim, I., Ko, B., & Li, W. (2015). Effects of improving teachers' content knowledge on teaching and student learning in physical education. *Research Quarterly for Exercise and Sport, 86*(2), 130–139.

Wilkinson, S. (1992). A training program for improving undergraduates' analytic skill in volleyball. *Journal of Teaching in Physical Education, 11*, 177–194.

Williams, L., & Rink, J. (2003). Chapter 5: Teacher competency using observational scoring rubrics. *Journal of Teaching in Physical Education, 22*, 555–572.

2 Skill analysis

Outcomes

- Understand the definitions of skill analysis.
- Identify different approaches to identify performance errors in skill analysis.
- Recognize and understand the components of the integrative biomechanical model of qualitative skill analysis and apply them to conduct skill analysis and how this model differentiates from other models.

Skill analysis

To be an effective physical education teacher or coach, one must develop competence in skill analysis. Skill analysis is an important tool for physical education teachers or coaches to have to improve students' or athletes' learning and performance. The importance for teachers or coaches to develop skill analysis competence is discussed in detail in Chapter 1. Some researchers have defined skill analysis as a process where discrepancies between the actual performance response observed and the ideal performance response are identified (Hoffman, 1977; Wilkinson, 1992). This definition focuses on the process of analysis. However, other components such as the preparation, evaluation, and intervention components are missing in the process of skill analysis. On the other hand, Knudson and Morrison (2002) have defined qualitative analysis/skill analysis as "the systematic observation and introspective judgment of the quality of human movement for the purpose of providing the most appropriate intervention to improve performance" (p. 4).

By integrating both definitions by Hoffman (1977), Wilkinson (1992), and Knudson and Morrison (2002), we define skill analysis as a process of preparing, observing, evaluating, and diagnosing skill performance by identifying correct and incorrect performance responses, and designing interventions to improve students' or athletes' skill performance based on the biomechanical model of the skills. This definition is more comprehensive and inclusive, which focuses on all aspects of skill analysis. First, teachers or coaches must be knowledgeable of the ideal performance response and all other capabilities needed for skill analysis through preparations. Second, teachers or coaches can evaluate and diagnose

DOI: 10.4324/9781003331964-3

students' or athletes' actual performance response based on their observations. What errors do students' or athletes' make? Why do those errors occur and how do those errors affect students' or athletes' performance based on biomechanically efficient and effective models of performance response? Finally, teachers or coaches can design developmentally appropriate interventions to correct their students' or athletes' performance errors.

Skill analysis can focus on either the technical or tactical aspects of a skill. When skill analysis focuses on the technical aspects of movement, it is called technical analysis. When skill analysis focuses on the tactical aspects of a skill, it is called tactical analysis. Skill analysis occurs when a teacher or coach systematically observes students' or athletes' game play and evaluates and diagnoses the appropriateness of their decision making in relation to the execution of their technical movement in a game context. For example, in a 2-versus-1 basketball offensive situation, the offensive player with the ball is pressured by the defender and tries to pass the ball to his or her teammate when the passing lane is closed out. This is an inappropriate decision making from the offensive player with the ball. The physical education teacher or coach can identify this tactical decision-making error and provide feedback to make sure that the offensive player with the ball only passes the ball when there is an open passing lane. In this book, we will use the term skill analysis, but mainly focus on technical analysis.

Four approaches to skill analysis

Since the 1970s, four different models or approaches have been proposed for qualitative analysis of human movements or sports skills, including sequential method, mechanical method, total body developmental stage method, and component sequence method (Knudson & Morrison, 2002). Those four approaches share a lot of commonalities in terms of the process of skill analysis from preparation or pre-observation planning to intervention. The key element that distinguishes those four approaches is how to identify skill errors.

The sequential method focuses on identifying errors through evaluation and diagnosis by comparing actual and mental desired/ideal skill performance, and then designing interventions to refine or advance the performance (Hay & Reid, 1988; Hoffman, 1977; Knudson & Morrison, 2002; Ward et al., 2021). The sequential method assumes that there is an ideal form, which is typically used by champion athletes (Hay & Reid, 1988; Knudson & Morrison, 2002).

The mechanical method detects skill errors by determining the differences between actual and desired performance based on biomechanical principles (Hay & Reid, 1988; Knudson & Morrison, 2002; Knudson, 2013). A desired skill performance is biomechanically efficient and effective. The biomechanical model of the skill is first established, where biomechanical principles underlying the efficiency and effectiveness of the skill performance and the relationships between those biomechanical principles and critical features of the skill are identified. Using this biomechanical deterministic model of the skill, teachers or coaches can evaluate students' or athletes' skill performance, identify their skill performance errors, and then develop interventions to fix their errors for better performance.

The total body developmental stage method focuses on error analysis through comparing movement features of actual skill performance and desired developmental stages, and then designing interventions to move students from one stage to more advanced stages. The total body developmental stage approach is a process measurement within the stage theory of motor skill development (Haubenstricker et al., 1983). It categorizes differential stages of skill development that describe process movements from one initial stage of the skill to subsequent more progressively mature stages (Haubenstricker et al., 1983). For example, Haubenstricker et al. (1983) identified five developmental stages of the overhand throwing skill with movement features at each of the five stages. In stage 1, a throwing performance consists of the movement features with no step or trunk rotation and a chopping arm movement. In stage 2, children perform throwing with their arm brought forward in transverse plane and may step forward. In stage 3, a throwing performance consists of an ipsilateral arm and leg movement. In stage 4, a throwing performance has movement features of contralateral step and striding forward but little or no rotation of the hips and spine. Finally, in stage 5, a throwing performance consists of stepping with wider contralateral step, trunk and hip rotation, and arm wind-up and follow through.

The Component Sequence approach focuses on error analysis through comparing skill progression features at each component of the skill of actual performance and desired performance and then develop interventions to fix those errors to move students from one skill progression to the next advanced progression at each component of the skill (Halverson & Roberton, 1984). The component sequence approach intends to measure the process or body movement variables that break down a skill into different components and each component contains different levels of progressions. It is assumed that changes in skill performance occur at the level of body components rather than the entire body. That is, component level changes can occur at different rates, at different times, and for different body components (Langendorfer & Roberton, 2002). For example, an overhand throwing skill can be broken into four body components: actions of step, trunk, humerus, and forearm, and each component has different levels of skill progressions. The component of step (Foot) action has four progressions: no step, homolateral step, contralateral and short step, and contralateral and long step. The body component of trunk (Pelvis-spine) action has three progressions: no trunk rotation, upper trunk rotation or total "block" rotation, and differentiated rotation. For the body component of forearm (Forward swing) action, it has three progressions: no forearm lag, forearm lag, and delayed forearm lag. The component of humerus (Upper arm) action during forward swing has three progressions: humerus oblique, humerus aligned but independent, and humerus lags (Halverson & Roberton, 1984).

All four approaches have their advantages and disadvantages. The sequential and biomechanical methods focus on critical features of the desired movements. They can be easily used by teachers or coaches in their teaching or coaching. The biomechanical method uses biomechanical principles to evaluate the efficiency and effectiveness of skill performances. However, a flaw in the sequential method is a lack of valid rationale for determining the ideal form of the skill (Hay & Reid, 1988; Knudson & Morrison, 2002). Both methods fail to consider developmental changes in movements as students or athletes mature. Those two methods may not detect specific changes in movements since they only rate those critical features as being present or absent in performance. The total body developmental stage and component sequence approaches integrate theories and research findings in motor development and learning and focus on critical features of the desired movements by incorporating developmental changes in movements. Both approaches assess movements qualitatively with precision. The total body approach is beneficial for teachers for them to analyze students' performance qualitatively. However, it has a ceiling effect since it assumes that individuals perform the same within the same stage. This approach is also difficult to detect minor changes in different components of the body movement such as trunk rotation, forearm lag, and humerus lag since it describes the movement components in one single stage (Haubenstricker et al., 1983). The component sequence method can detect minor changes in body movement patterns and allow researchers to analyze movement profiles more precisely during the performance (Lorson & Goodway, 2008; Langendorfer & Roberton, 2002). However, the disadvantage of the component sequence approach is the difficulty for teachers to assess the trunk, humerus, and forearm components in real time while teaching without use of videotape analysis. It is almost impossible and impractical for teachers to differentiate trunk, humerus, or forearm components in real time while teaching since those components must be observed in different angles. Both the total body and component sequence methods have not been widely used in sports coaching.

In this book, we use the biomechanical approach to conduct skill analysis. Critical elements/features of a skill based on biomechanical principles will be identified and recorded in a skill analysis observation sheet according to three phases of skill execution. Tables 2.1 through 2.8 present some examples for skill analysis observation sheets. The first column consists of three phases of skill execution. The second column consists of critical elements/features of a skill, which are derived based on the biomechanical principles. For the third column, the biomechanical principles in relation to those critical features are described. For the fourth column, a teacher or coach will rate students' or players' performance response by indicating whether those critical elements or features are present or not in their performance. The last column is where a teacher or coach can provide some detailed comments with regards to those corresponding elements. For example, if a student or player had a follow-

Table 2.1 Skill analysis sheet for skipping

Phase	Critical elements	Bio-mechanical explanations	Present (yes/no)	Comments
Preparation	1 Feet shoulder-width apart 2 Facing the direction 3 Back straight 4 Eyes forward 5 Arms and hands naturally on sides			
Execution/ Follow through	1 Step forward and hop on same foot 2 Step forward on other foot, hop on same foot 3 Springlike action on hops 4 Swing arms to chest levels in opposition 5 Land lightly on balls of feet			

Table 2.2 Skill analysis sheet for volleyball overhead passing (set)

Phase	Critical elements	Bio-mechanical explanations	Present? (yes/no)	Comments
Preparation	1 Back Straight 2 Eyes on ball 3 Knees bent 4 Feet shoulder width apart 5 Face target			
Execution	1 Head looking up 2 Spread fingers 3 Hands make triangle right above head 4 Arms bent 5 Elbow up and out 6 Extended legs and arms 7 Contact with fingers on side of ball with both hands simultaneously 8 Flick your wrists out near the end of your arm extension			
Follow through	1 Rainbow follow-through			

Table 2.3 Skill analysis sheet for volleyball forearm passing

Phase	Critical elements	Bio-mechanical explanations	Present? (yes/no)	Comments
Preparation	1 Feet shoulder width apart 2 Eyes on ball 3 Back Straight 4 Knees bent 5 Hands cupped, thumbs together 6 Body aligned with the target 7 Arms extended with flat forearm platform			
Execution	1 Move under the ball 2 Bend legs more 3 Arms straighten when ball contacts forearm 4 Make contact with forearm flat platform 5 Lift with legs while making contact			
Follow through	1 Arms guide ball to target			

Table 2.4 Skill analysis sheet for volleyball underhand serving

Phase	Critical elements	Bio-mechanical explanations	Present? (yes/no)	Comments
Preparation	1 Face target 2 Back straight 3 Knees bent with opposite foot slightly in front of "serving arm" foot 4 Non-serving arm extended in front of body palm up with ball resting in palm			
Execution	1 Swing serving arm back 2 Step forward with opposite foot 3 Shift weight to the front 4 Swing arm forward 5 Keep hitting arm straight 6 Contact the bottom of the ball with heel of hand 7 Hit ball off hand			
Follow through	1 Swing through ball 2 Keep hitting arm up facing target			

Table 2.5 Skill analysis sheet for soccer shooting

Phase	Critical elements	Bio-mechanical explanations	Present? (yes/no)	Comments
Preparation	1 Feet shoulder width 2 Face target 3 Knees bent 4 Back straight 5 Eyes on target			
Execution	1 Approach to the ball 2 Elongated stride prior to planting foot beside the ball 3 Plant the non kicking foot beside ball 4 Shift weight to non kicking foot 5 Bring kicking foot backward with knee bent 6 Swing kicking foot forward straightening the knee 7 Square foot to ball 8 Make contact with ball			
Follow through	1 Kick through the ball 2 Land on kicking foot first then non kicking foot			

Table 2.6 Skill analysis sheet for team handball overhand passing

Phase	Critical elements	Bio-mechanical explanations	Present? (yes/no)	Comments
Preparation	1 Feet shoulder width apart 2 Face target, 3 Back straight 4 Knees slightly bent 5 Ball in both hands at chest level 6 Eyes on target			
Execution	1 Step forward to target with the opposite foot 2 Rotate trunk 3 Bring throwing arm back to ear, with elbow at shoulder 4 Arm in L shape 5 Opposite arm aimed at target 6 Rotate trunk forward 7 Shift body weight to front foot bring arm forward 8 Release ball at shoulder level 9 Bring non-throwing arm back			
Follow through	1 Follow through to the opposite leg			

Table 2.7 Skill analysis sheet for swimming freestyle

Phase	Critical elements	Bio-mechanical explanations	Present? (yes/no)	Comments
Preparation	1 Position your body parallel to the bottom of the pool			
	2 Head centered and cocked about 45 degrees forward			
	3 Eyes focused ahead and on the bottom of the pool			
	4 Dominant arm on side			
	5 Opposite arm straight and forward			
Execution	1 Lift right (dominant) arm out of the water			
	2 Elbow bent and pointed to the ceiling			
	3 Extend right arm and reach forward			
	4 Keep fingers together			
	5 Make a slight "cup" with your hand			
	6 Roll your right shoulder forward and down			
	7 Twist and pivot body to right side at 120 degree			
	8 Pull opposite arm down through the water until parallel with your side			
	9 Curve your hand back inward toward your belly button and out by hip as hand "pulls" on the water and exits			
	10 Lift left arm out of the water			
	11 Elbow bent and pointed to the ceiling			
	12 Extend left arm and reach forward			
	13 Keep fingers together			
	14 Make a slight "cup" with your hand			
	15 Roll your left shoulder forward and down			
	16 Twist and pivot body to left side at 120 degree			
	17 Pull opposite arm down through the water until parallel with your side			
	18 Curve your left hand back inward toward your belly button and out by hip as hand "pulls" on the water and exits			
	19 Lift right arm out of the water			
	20 Elbow bent and pointed to the ceiling			
	21 Place your ear on left shoulder and your cheek in the water,			
	22 Use mouth to breathe in			
	23 Breathe out all of your air through nose under water			
	24 Points your toes			
	25 "Flutter kick" your feet just below the surface of the water			
Follow through				

Table 2.8 Skill analysis sheet for swimming butterfly

Phase	Critical elements	Bio-mechanical explanations	Present? (yes/no)	Comments
Preparation	1 Place yourself laterally in the water 2 Arms extended straight above head with shoulder width apart 3 Legs extended in back of you			
Execution	1 Pull hands towards body in a semicircular motion 2 Palms facing outwards 3 Push palms backward through the water, along your sides and past your hips 4 Sweep both arms out of the water simultaneously 5 Throw them forward into the starting position 6 Palms facing outwards with thumbs entering the water first 7 Dolphin kicks with both legs			
Follow through				

through movement, however, the follow-through movement is not complete. The teacher or coach can check yes but indicate incomplete follow through. Or the teacher or coach can check no but indicate that the student or player did not have a complete follow through, or in a game context, the student or player did not need to have a complete follow through motion.

In general, an execution of a sport skill can be divided into three phases: preparation, execution, and follow-through. The preparation phase includes all the elements of body parts in preparation for executing a movement. The execution phase refers to the initiation and end of body parts to execute a movement. The follow-through phase is to continue body motion to its conclusion such as cushioning the body after landing or extending the body motion for power. Those three phases typically occur in a discrete skill such as triple jump, kicking a soccer ball, throwing, and hitting a ball, which has a definite beginning and end. However, for a continuous, repetitive skill such as running, skipping, and swimming, the last two phases of execution and follow-through are combined since they have no clear end and it is difficult to separate the movement elements of those two phases. Then a teacher or coach will conduct systematic observation of skill performance. Through observations, he or she will identify the discrepancies between actual and desired performance responses among his or her students or players and use biomechanical principles to understand why the errors occur and how those errors affect their performance. Finally, a teacher or coach can design developmentally appropriate interventions to refine or advance students' or athletes' performance.

Models of qualitative analysis

Different models of qualitative analysis have been proposed by scholars since the 1970s.

In the following section, four major models will be briefly described since our proposed model in this book integrates the major components of those four models. In the final section, we will describe our model of skill analysis.

In 1976, Arend and Higgins proposed a comprehensive model of human movement analysis from an interdisciplinary approach. Numerous kinesiology subdisciplines are integrated in the plan for analysis, including biomechanics, motor development, motor learning, physiology, physical education pedagogy, etc. This model has three steps: pre-observation, observation, and post-observation. The pre-observation stage involves the amassing of prerequisite information or content knowledge for teaching and setting the foundation for observation, evaluation, and diagnosis in the observation and post-observation stages. The prerequisite information consists of the description and analysis of the movement, the movement environment, essential needs of the performer, essential features of the movement, and the performer. The description and analysis of the movement and the environment has a three-order decomposition. The first-order decomposition is to conduct a descriptive analysis of the movement (i.e., goals, types), classify the environment (open versus closed), and break the movement into general parts or phases. The second-order decomposition quantitatively or qualitatively provides more specific descriptions of the movements in each part or phase. The third-order decomposition provides a rationale for the movement through the identification of important correlates of each phase of the movement such as biomechanical principles and others. The observation stage is to observe and record "what happened" during the performance in a systematic approach. The post-observation stage is to conduct comparative evaluation and analysis of observed performance based on the gained information in the first two stages and then provide feedback for the performer to improve performance.

In the 1980s, Hay and his colleagues proposed another comprehensive model of qualitative analysis (Hay, 1984; Hay & Reid, 1982, 1988). This model consists of four steps. The first step is to develop a biomechanical

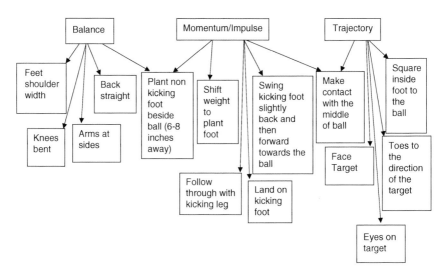

Figure 2.1 Biomechanical model of soccer in-step passing.

model of the skill. Based on the purpose of the skill, biomechanical factors that determine the skill performance are identified. For example, the purpose of a basketball foul shot is to project the basketball into the basket. To accomplish the goal of this task, students must generate sufficient power/momentum for distance and a trajectory for accuracy. Figure 2.1 illustrates a biomechanical model of soccer in-step passing. Abendroth-Smith and his colleagues (Abendroth-Smith et al., 1996; Abendroth-Smith, & Kras, 1999) expanded this biomechanical model of qualitative analysis to physical education teaching by integrating the skill levels of students (beginner, intermediate, and advanced) and phases of movements (pre-execution, execution, and post-execution) for skill analysis. It is called Biomechanically based Observation and Analysis for Teachers (BBOAT).

The second step is to observe performance and identify performance errors. Several recommendations are provided by Hay and Reid (1988) on how to conduct performance observations, including the usage of multiple senses, vantage points, number of observations, observational settings, consideration of fatigues and learners' skill and age levels, etc. The third step is to prioritize the errors. In step three, teachers or coaches examine the relationships among those identified errors, rank their importance, and determine the order in which those errors will be fixed. It is very important to identify the roots that cause each of those errors. In some cases, one error is caused by another error. When you fix the other error, this error will be fixed accordingly. The final step is to provide instructions for the performer to correct those performance errors. During this step, teachers or coaches will design developmentally appropriate interventions to fix those errors based on the involved biomechanical principles. This step is critical since inappropriate interventions will not result in any improvement in students' or athletes' skill performance.

In 1990, McPherson proposed another comprehensive model of qualitative analysis based on the previous biomechanical models (Knudson & Morrison, 2002; McPherson, 1990). The McPherson model of qualitative analysis consists of four steps: pre-observation, observation, diagnosis, and remediation. This model is like the Hay and Reid (1982, 1988) model, but provides more thorough discussions of each of the four steps in a systematical way and connects biomechanics with critical features of the skill (Knudson & Morrison, 2002). In 2002, Knudson and Morrison proposed an integrated model of qualitative analysis for movement (Knudson & Morrison, 2002). This model consists of four components: preparation, observation, evaluation/diagnosis, and intervention. The first component of preparation is a continuous process where teachers or coaches build a prerequisite knowledge base for observation, evaluation/diagnosis, and intervention. The prerequisite knowledge base consists of three major areas: knowledge about the activity or movement, knowledge about the performer, and knowledge about effective instruction. The second component of this model is observation, which is to use effective observational strategies to observe and record the performer's skill performance. Through observation, teachers or coaches gather information about students' or athletes' skill performance. The third component of this model is evaluation and diagnostic. After gathering students' or athletes' skill performance, teachers or coaches will use their prerequisite knowledge to conduct evaluation and diagnostic of their skill performance. Teachers or coaches will identify the strengths and weaknesses in their students' or athletes' skill performance by comparing their actual performance with the biomechanically efficient and effective form of the skill. This will lay a foundation for teachers or coaches to develop interventions to fix errors, thus improving skill performance. The last component of this model is intervention. Based on evaluation and diagnostic of students' skill performance, teachers or coaches select effective intervention strategies to fix their students' or athletes' errors to increase performance. Those interventions can include vision aids, feedback, physical assistance, and practices, etc.

By integrating the components of each of four models, we propose an integrated biomechanical model of Qualitative Skill Analysis as shown in Figure 2.2. This model provides conceptual guidance on how to conduct skill analysis. The IBMQSA is mostly like integrative model of qualitative analysis. Both models consist of the same four components: preparation, observation, evaluation/diagnosis, and intervention. There are two significant differences between the IBMQSA and integrative model of qualitative analysis. The first difference is that the IBMQSA uses a biomechanical approach to identify skill errors and provide a rationale for analysis and interventions. The second difference is that all kinesiology subdisciplines are fully and systematically integrated into the entire model, including biomechanics,

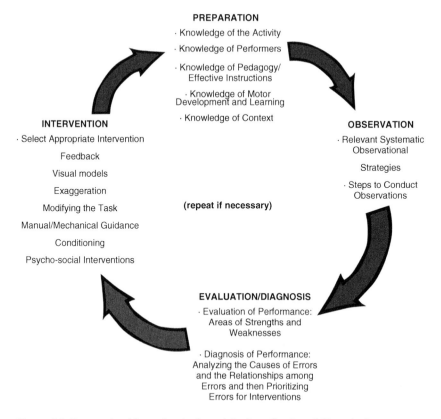

Figure 2.2 Integrative biomechanical model of qualitative skill analysis.

Source: Adapted from *Qualitative diagnosis of human movement: Improving performance in sport and exercise* by Duane V. Knudson (2013). Copyright permission obtained.

motor development, motor learning, physiology, physical education pedagogy, etc. The first component of preparation is informed by the framework
of content knowledge and pedagogical content knowledge and integrates
numerous kinesiology subdisciplines. The prerequisite knowledge base consists of six major areas: knowledge of performers, knowledge of pedagogy,
knowledge of contexts, knowledge of skills/movement, knowledge of biomechanics, and knowledge of motor development and learning. All the
kinesiology sub-disciplinary knowledge is integrated in the evaluation/diag-
nosis of skills and development of interventions to improve skill performance.

Summary

Effective physical education teachers or coaches must possess competence in
skill analysis, which is an important tool for them to improve students' or
athletes' learning and performance. Four different approaches have been

developed to identify performance errors: sequential method, mechanical method, total body developmental stage method, and component sequence method. Those four approaches share some commonalities, and each approach has its advantages and disadvantages. Over the past 30 years, scholars have proposed various models to conduct qualitative analysis of human movements or sports skills. The IBMQSA consists of four components: preparation, observation, evaluation/diagnosis, and intervention. It uses a biomechanical approach to identify skill errors and provide a rationale for analysis and interventions. All kinesiology subdisciplines are fully and systematically integrated into the entire model, including biomechanics, motor development, motor learning, physiology, physical education pedagogy, etc. Especially, the preparation component is informed by the framework of content knowledge and pedagogical content knowledge.

Questions for reflection

- What is the definition of skill analysis?
- What are four different approaches to identifying performance errors in skill analysis?
- What is an integrated biomechanical model of qualitative skill analysis? How does this model differentiate from other qualitative analysis models?
- What are the four components of integrated biomechanical model of qualitative skill analysis?

References

Abendroth-Smith, J., & Kras, J. (1999). More BBOAT: The volleyball spike. *Journal of Physical Education, Recreation, and Dance, 70*(3), 56–59.

Abendroth-Smith, J., Kras, J., & Strand, B. (1996). Get aboard the BBOAT: Biomechanically based observation and analysis for teachers. *Journal of Physical Education, Recreation, and Dance, 67*(8), 20–23.

Arend, S., & Higgins, J. R. (1976). A strategy for the classification, subjective analysis and observation of human movement. *Journal of Human Movement Studies, 2*(1), 36–52.

Halverson, L. E., & Roberton, M. A. (1984). *Developing children – Their changing movement: A guide for teachers.* Philadelphia, PA: Lippincott Williams & Wilkins.

Haubenstricker, J. L., Brantas, C. F., & Seefeldt, V. D. (1983). *Standards of performance for throwing and catching.* East Lansing, Michigan: American Society for the Psychology of Sprot and Physical Activity.

Hay, J. G. (1984). The development of deterministic models for qualitative analysis. In R. Shapiro and J. R. Marett (Eds.), *Proceedings: Second national symposium on teaching kinesiology and biomechanics in sports* (pp. 71–83). Colorado Springs, CO: NASPE.

Hay, J. G., & Reid, J. G. (1982). *The anatomical and mechanical bases of human motion.* Englewood Cliffs, NJ: Prentice-Hall.

Hay, J. G., & Reid, J. G. (1988). *Anatomy, mechanics, and human motion* (2nd ed.). Englewood Cliffs, NJ: Prentice-Hall.

Hoffman, S. J. (1977). Competency based training in skill analysis. In R. E. Stadulis (Eds.), *Research and practice in physical education* (pp. 3–12). Champaign, IL: Human Kinetics.

Knudson, D. V. (2013). *Qualitative diagnosis of human movement: Improving performance in sport and exercise.* Champaign, IL: Human Kinetics.

Knudson, D. V., & Morrison, C. S. (2002). *Qualitative analysis of human movement* (2nd ed.). Champaign, IL: Human Kinetics.

Langendorfer, S., & Roberton, M. A. (2002). Developmental profiles in overarm throwing: searching for "attractors", "stages", and "constraints". In J. E. Clark & J. H. Humphrey (Eds.), *Motor development: Research and review: Vol. 2.* (pp. 1–25). Reston, VA: NASPE Publications.

Lorson, K., & Goodway, J. D. (2008). Gender differences in throwing form of children ages 6–8 years during a throwing game. *Research Quarterly for Exercise and Sport*, 79(2), 174–182.

McPherson, M. N. (1990). A systematic approach to skill analysis. *Sports Science Periodical on Research and Technology in Sport*, 11(1), 1–10.

Wilkinson, S. (1992). A training program for improving undergraduates' analytic skill in volleyball. *Journal of Teaching in Physical Education*, 11, 177–194.

Ward, P., Ayvazo, S., Dervent, F., Iserbyt, P., Kim, I., & Li, W. (2021). Skill analysis for teachers: Considerations for physical education teacher education. *Journal of Physical Education, Recreation & Dance*, 92(2), 15–21.

Section 2

Preparation

This section focuses on the first component of the Integrative Biomechanical Model of Qualitative Skill Analysis Preparation, which has six chapters. Chapter 3 introduces the definition of preparation and discusses five major knowledge bases for the teacher or coach to possess, including knowledge of performers, knowledge of sports skill, knowledge of the biomechanical model of the skill, knowledge of effective instructions, and knowledge of motor learning and control. Chapter 4 defines sports analysis, skill, technique, and tactics, discusses the similarities and differences among skills, techniques, and tactics, and introduces steps to successfully conduct sports analysis. Chapter 5 focuses on understanding movement preparation, specifically, a cognitive process that precedes the production of a skillful movement and introduces the theoretical models and behavioral measures of movement preparation, as well as the factors that influence movement preparation. Chapter 6 focuses on understanding the control mechanism underlying skilled movements and two motor control mechanisms are introduced. Chapter 7 focuses on understanding motor learning from the learner's perspective. Two models of stages of learning will be introduced. Different kinds of performance measures are discussed to help with detecting motor learning. Chapter 8 defines what is task progressions, introduces the concept of task and task development, discusses factors that affect task complexity, and how to design task progressions.

DOI: 10.4324/9781003331964-4

3 Preparation

DOI: 10.4324/9781003331964-5

Outcomes

What is preparation?

- What are major knowledge bases that teachers or coaches need to possess for qualitative skill analysis?
- What is the biomechanical model of skills?
- What is instruction?
- What is demonstration?
- What is feedback? What are the different types of feedback?

Knowledge of performers

Students or athletes come to play sports with different entry characteristics. Those characteristics include cultural, social, and educational backgrounds, age, athletic skill levels, gender, motivation, attitudes, cognition, and experiences, etc. Knowledge of those entry characteristics can facilitate teachers or coaches to plan effective instructions and pedagogies accordingly, which can significantly affect students' or athletes' learning and performance outcomes. The more knowledge of students or athletes, the better teachers or coaches can evaluate and analyze their skills and design interventions to improve their performance outcomes. For example, in physical education, teachers present instructions differently and use different methods and pedagogies to teach a sport skill to 3rd graders than 8th graders since they are in different stages of cognitive development and have different playing experiences in sports. For 3rd graders, physical education teachers can present the whole skill with diagrams, videos, or physical demonstrations and focus on one to two critical elements at a time during their practices. For 8th graders, they can present the whole skill with diagrams, videos, or physical demonstrations, but empower students with opportunities to self-teach themselves using a discovery learning method during their practices. Knowing the skill levels and experiences of students or athletes will help teachers or coaches anticipate what potential errors they will make in their performance and potential intervention methods to use to fix those errors. It will also help teachers or coaches to design initial practices to improve students' or athletes' skill performances through developmentally appropriate and progressive practices.

Knowledge of sports skills

An extensive knowledge of the activity or skill is critical to conduct a good analysis. First, teachers or coaches must know what is the goal of the activity or skill? For example, the goal for long jump is to project the body for a long distance. Understanding the goal of the activity or skill can help teachers or coaches identify biomechanics underlying the activity or skill and develop practices to achieve the goal. In the case of long jump, momentum and trajectory are two critical biomechanics that will determine how far students or athletes can jump. To generate momentum, teachers or coaches can design practices to increase the speed of running approach and leg power of students or athletes. To produce the optimal trajectory for distance, teachers or coaches can focus on the angle of take-off to be between 15 and 27 degrees.

Secondly, teachers or coaches must know the elements of how to perform the activity or skill. To perform an activity or a skill, students or athletes must utilize different body parts in a sequential manner to produce a biomechanically efficient and effective performance. The key features of an activity or a skill are called critical elements, which are necessary to produce optimal performance (Knudson & Morrison, 2002). They define a good form which is biomechanically efficient and effective and should be the focus in the qualitative analysis of the activity or skill. Table 3.1 presents an example of critical elements of soccer in-step passing skill. A solid knowledge base of the critical elements of an activity or a skill will help teachers or coaches identify errors in their athletes' or students' performance and design practices to correct those errors.

Table 3.1 Critical elements of soccer in-step passing

Phase	Critical elements
Preparation	1 Feet shoulder width
	2 Face target
	3 Back straight
	4 Arms at side
	5 Knees bent
	6 Eyes on target
Execution	1 Approaching to the ball
	2 Arms swing in opposition
	3 Plant non kicking foot beside ball (6–8 inches away)
	4 Toes to the direction of the target
	5 Shift weight to plant foot
	6 Swing kicking foot slightly back and then forward towards the ball
	7 Square foot to ball
	8 Make contact with the middle of the ball
Follow through	1 Follow through with kicking leg
	2 Land on kicking foot

Source: Copyright permission obtained.

Knowledge of the biomechanical model of skills

The execution of critical elements of a skill is critical to achieve an optimal performance. The existence of those critical elements has important bio-mechanical bases. Abendroth-Smith et al. (1996) proposed a biomechanical model, which describes the biomechanical basis of the critical elements of a sport skill. In this model, major important biomechanical principles in rela-tion to the goal of the skill and the relationships between those biomechanical principles and the critical elements are clearly identified. Figure 3.1 is an example of a biomechanical model of soccer in-step passing.

Biomechanics is an area of study of the application of mechanical knowledge, principles, and methods to the structure and function of the human body (Kreighbaum & Barthels, 1996). The biomechanical principles and laws of motion control human movement, which have important appli-cations to sports skill performances. Those biomechanical principles and laws of motion can often be transferrable to sports with a similar purpose. Poor biomechanics lead to poor techniques, which results in inferior performance outcomes. Most of the top-class athletes use superior techniques, which are based on sound bio-mechanical principles.

A knowledge of the biomechanical model can help teachers or coaches distinguish between mechanically correct movements and those that are not. Any violation of these biomechanical principles and laws of motion are often the cause of errors. This makes it possible for teachers or coaches to deal with the mechanisms of human motion to accurately identify errors and develop interventions to fix those errors for skill development and improvement. This process where teachers or coaches apply biomechanical principles for error detection forms the basis of skill analysis. For example, when practicing

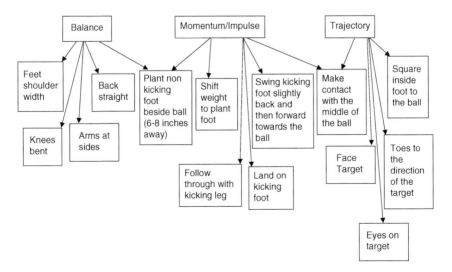

Figure 3.1 Biomechanical model of soccer in-step passing.

soccer in-step passing, a student or an athlete kicks the ball off to the right side of his or her teammate. If teachers or coaches have a good knowledge of the biomechanical model in Figure 3.1, they will be able to use the bio-mechanical principle of trajectory to quickly identify three possible technical reasons that cause the error. One possible cause is that this student or athlete contacts the right side of the ball rather than the middle of the ball. The other one is that this student or athlete fails to square foot to the soccer ball. Another one is that this student or athlete does not keep the toes of the supporting leg pointed toward the ball. After understanding the potential causes of the performance error, then teachers or coaches can design corresponding interventions to fix the error based on the specific deficiency in the student's or athlete's performance. If teachers or coaches have an in-depth knowledge of biomechanical models for all skills in the sports they teach or coach, the quality of teaching or coaching will increase. As a result, students or athletes will improve their learning and performances.

Knowledge of effective instructions

In the teaching or coaching process, two important instructional factors affecting teaching or coaching effectiveness are effective task instruction and demonstration and effective feedback.

Effective task instruction and demonstration

Task instruction and demonstration is a critical skill for teachers or coaches to have for successful teaching or coaching. Teachers or coaches must be able to represent a task to students or athletes in a clear, accurate, and comprehensible way for them to learn. Task instruction is defined as "Teacher is verbally describing to the students how to do a skill or using a verbal prompt to direct students in attempting a skill or activity" (Hawkins & Wiegand, 1989, p. 279). An effective task instruction should meet the following five criteria: (1) It should be accurate and concise. Accurate and concise information is key for students or athletes to learn to successfully perform a skill. Otherwise, students or athletes will make many errors because of inaccurate instruction, which leads to inferior performance outcomes. Too lengthy and/or irrelevant information can overwhelm students or athletes who would be lost and miss the key information for successful learning. (2) It should include the critical elements of the skill. The successful execution of those critical elements is crucial for successful performance. Teachers or coaches should always start with major critical elements to help students or athletes grasp the whole picture of the skill and then gradually focus on refining the specific aspects of the skill through deliberate practices with constant and congruent feedback. (3) It should contain analogies or metaphors. Using analogies or metaphors makes instruction fun and interesting to learn, easy to understand and memorize, and relevant to students' or athletes' real lives. (4) It should be developmentally appropriate for students' or athletes' ability levels and experiences. Students or athletes vary in their abilities, have a differentiated rate of skill learning, are at different stages of physical, cognitive, and emotional developments, and have different levels of experiences. Therefore, when teachers or coaches give instruction, they must take those elements into consideration. Finally, (5) It should have a clear and concise task statement with situation, behavior, a goal, and criteria. When teachers or coaches give a clear task statement, athletes or students know exactly what to do, how to do it, and what to accomplish. This will increase the opportunities for students or athletes to successfully perform the task, thus improving their performance.

Demonstration is defined as "modeling desired performance executed by teacher, student(s), and/or visual aids" (Rink, 2006, p. 372). It helps students or athletes visually understand the instruction; therefore, they will know what to focus on during practice and how to successfully perform the skill. Teachers or coaches often demonstrate a skill physically by themselves. This requires them to have an excellent skill performance since it models desired performance. Teachers or coaches can use their students or athletes to demonstrate a skill. Using students or athletes for demonstration can empower them with a leadership opportunity and increase their self-esteem. This can also potentially help create a positive student-centered or athlete-centered team culture. Teachers or coaches can also use other visual aids to demonstrate a skill, including iPhone, iPad, videos, task cards, pictures, and diagrams etc. With the availability of current advanced technology, teachers or coaches have easy access to performance videos of top-flight athletes. Teachers can play those video clips on a projector screen in a gym. Coaches can play those video clips on their iPhones or iPad during coaching. Teachers or coaches have choices to select one or two different ways to demonstrate a skill based on their own performance capabilities and students' or athletes' abilities and backgrounds.

Effective feedback

During and after practices, teachers or coaches often need to increase students' or athletes' motivation, reinforce the correct performance, or remediate the errors by providing feedback. Skill-related feedback is the information that teachers or coaches provide to students or athletes, with a goal of increasing their performances by reducing the discrepancies between the actual and desired performances (Hattie & Timperley, 2007) of students or athletes. Feedback from teachers or coaches plays an important role in students' or athletes' skill development. Feedback can be classified in many ways based on the form, type, referent, target, and timing of feedback. The form, target, and time of teacher feedback are generally verbal versus non-verbal, individual versus group, and immediate or delayed, respectively. Feedback can also be classified as general versus specific, positive versus negative, knowledge of performance versus knowledge of results, or corrective based on what and how information is provided to students or athletes. Please see Table 3.2 for examples of different types of feedback.

Table 3.2 Examples for various types of feedback

Types of feedback	Definition	Examples
General feedback	The information provided by coaches or teachers is very general.	Good job.
Specific feedback	The information provided by coaches or teachers is specific with details with regard to athletes' or students' behaviors or skill performances.	Well done. You extended your elbow!
Positive feedback	The information provided by coaches or teachers is encouraging and supportive.	Great. What a perfect take off!
Negative feedback	The information provided by coaches or teachers is negative.	Your swing is bad.
Corrective feedback	The information provided by coaches or teachers is to correct athletes' or students' errors in their performances.	Next time, please rotate your shoulders clockwise
Knowledge of results	The information provided by coaches or teachers is to focus on the product or outcome of skill performances.	Your ball landed out of the boundary.
Knowledge of performance	The information provided by coaches or teachers is to focus on the elements of skills for future performance improvements.	Make sure to swing all the way to have a good follow through.

Researchers have investigated the effects of teacher feedback on student learning and performance in physical education (Behets, 1997; Cohen et al., 2012; Fredenburg et al., 2001; Mouratidis et al., 2008; Rikard, 1991, 1992; Yerg, 1981). A Review study by Lee et al. (1993) showed that the effects of teacher feedback on student learning and performance were inconclusive. Various factors such as the amount, quality, timing, and types of feedback can contribute to the inconclusive findings (Lee et al., 1993). However, based on anecdotal evidence, to improve students' or athletes' skill performance, feedback from teachers or coaches must be positive, specific, and congruent, which focuses on correcting errors in their performance. Sometimes, teachers or coaches can provide general feedback such as good job to motivate their students or athletes to be more engaged in their practices and game plays.

Knowledge of motor learning and control

Skill acquisition is by nature a process of changing behavior to improve motor performance, during which teachers or coaches are the facilitators of behavioral changes. The study of Motor Learning and Control (MLC) has been focused on uncovering the principles of learning and control of skilled movements using various methods to capture, assess, and change motor behavior. From inside out and outside in, MLC theories embrace the interaction among factors of learner, task, and environment in shaping various motor behaviors, which provides a foundation for developing behavioral interventions. Therefore, teachers or coaches should be equipped with the knowledge of MLC so that their knowledge of students, skills, and biomechanics (introduced in Chapters 9–13) can be integrated as one to facilitate skill acquisition in their practice of teaching and coaching. Chapters 5–7 will further discuss MLC theories and their applications in skill analysis.

Summary

This chapter focuses on the first component of the Integrative Biomechanical Model of Qualitative Skill Analysis: preparation. To prepare for qualitative skill analysis, teachers or coaches must possess five major knowledge bases, including knowledge of performers, knowledge of the activity, knowledge of the biomechanical model of skills, knowledge of effective instructions, and knowledge of motor learning and control. Those knowledge bases are critical for teachers or coaches to detect students' or athletes' performance errors and develop appropriate interventions to fix them, thus improving their learning and performances.

Questions for reflection

- What is the definition of preparation?
- What are the main five knowledge bases that coaches or teachers must possess to prepare for qualitative skill analysis? Why are they important for coaches or teachers to prepare for qualitative skill analysis?
- Please provide a specific example for seven different types of feedback.
- Please map out a biomechanical model of a specific sport skill.

References

Abendroth-Smith, J., Kras, J., & Strand, B. (1996). Get aboard the BBOAT: Biomechanically based observation and analysis for teachers. *Journal of Physical Education, Recreation, and Dance, 67*(8), 20–23.

Behets, D. (1997). Comparison of more and less effective teaching behaviors in secondary physical education. *Teaching and Teacher Education, 13*(2), 215–224.

Cohen, R., Goodway, J. D., & Lidor, R. (2012). The effectiveness of aligned developmental feedback on the overhand throw in third-grade students. *Physical Education & Sport Pedagogy, 17*(5), 525–541.

Fredenburg, K. B., Lee, A. M., & Solmon, M. (2001). The effects of augmented feedback on students' perceptions and performance. *Research Quarterly for Exercise and Sport, 72*(3), 232–242.

Hattie, J., & Timperley, H. (2007). The power of feedback. *Review of Educational Research, 77*(1), 81–112.

Hawkins, A., & Wiegand, R. (1989). West Virginia University teaching evaluation system and feedback taxonomy. In P. Darst, R. Zakrajsek, & V. Mancini (Eds.), *Analyzing physical education and sport Instruction* (pp. 277–293). Champaign, IL: Human Kinetics.

Knudson, D. V., & Morrison, C. S. (2002). *Qualitative analysis of human movement* (2nd ed.). Champaign, IL: Human Kinetics.

Kreighbaum, E., & Barthels, K. M. (1996). *Biomechanics: A qualitative approach for studying human movement* (4th ed.). Boston, MA: Allyn & Bacon.

Lee, A. M., Keh, N. C., & Magill, R. A. (1993). Instructional effects of teacher feedback in physical education. *Journal of Teaching in Physical Education, 12*(3), 228–243.

Mouratidis, A., Vansteenkiste, M., Lens, W., & Sideridis, G. (2008). The motivating role of positive feedback in sport and physical education: Evidence for a motivational model. *Journal of Sport & Exercise Psychology, 30*(2), 240–268.

Rikard, G. L. (1991). The short term relationship of teacher feedback and student practices. *Journal of Teaching in Physical Education, 10*(3), 275–285.

Rikard, G. L. (1992). The relationship of teachers' task refinement and feedback to students' practice success. *Journal of Teaching in Physical Education, 11*(4), 349–357.

Rink, J. E. (2006). *Teaching physical education for learning* (5th ed.). Boston, MA: McGraw-Hill.

Yerg, B. J. (1981). Reflections on the use of the RTE model in physical education. *Research Quarterly for Exercise and Sport, 52*(1), 38–47.

4 Sport analysis
Knowledge of Sports Skills

Outcomes

- Define what is sports analysis.
- Understand the similarities and differences between techniques, skills, and tactics.
- Identify the four components of sports analysis.
- Conduct sports analysis.

There is a saying that goes "Do not talk about things we know nothing about". This is very much true when we apply this maxim to teaching or coaching sports. Teachers or coaches must obtain all the knowledge related to a sport to effectively teach or coach it to students or athletes. For example, if you are going to teach basketball, you need to be familiar with basketball history, culture, rules, techniques and tactics, equipment and facility, and progressive practices that can advance students or athletes from one level to the next. When we package all the information together into a database, we produce a knowledge package. This knowledge package contains common content knowledge that teachers or coaches need to effectively teach or coach a sport to students or athletes. The process of developing the knowledge package is what we call sports analysis. In this chapter, you will learn how to develop a knowledge package through conducting sports analysis.

Sports analysis and components

Being knowledgeable of all the components in a sport is a critical skill that teachers or coaches need to develop to lay a foundation for teaching or coaching effectiveness. Sports analysis is the process of systematically identifying, analyzing, and sequencing all the components in a sport necessary for effective teaching or coaching. There are three main purposes for conducting sports analysis. The first purpose is to identify, define, and describe all the components for a sport that teachers or coaches need to know for effective teaching or coaching. The second purpose is to analyze and identify appropriate progressive practices to advance students or athletes from one level to

DOI: 10.4324/9781003331964-6

the next level. The last purpose is to identify all the games and activities that can be used to develop teamwork and maximize students' or athletes' motivation for better learning and performance.

The components in sport analysis consist of five domains: (1) physiological training and conditioning, (2) background knowledge, (3) psychomotor skills (techniques and tactics), (4) progressive practices, and (5) psycho-social concepts. In the following sections, the five components will be described in detail with specific examples to help teachers or coaches learn how to conduct sports analysis.

Physiological training and conditioning

Physical training and conditioning are critical to achieving successful performance in sports. As a teacher or coach, you need to possess the essential knowledge and skills related to physical training and conditioning. A typical complete physical conditioning workout consists of three main components: 5- to 10-minute warm-up, main conditioning training, and 5- to 10-minute cool-down. The main conditioning training usually consists of weightlifting and aerobic exercises to develop muscular strength and endurance and cardiovascular capacity. For warm-up and cool-down exercises, they can be general warm-up, cool-down, and stretching exercises or sports-specific warm-up and stretching exercises. General warm-up and cool-down exercises can be slow walking, fast walking, jogging, or running while sports-specific warm-up may focus on some basic skill practices such as shooting, passing, and lay-ups in basketball.

There are four different types of stretching exercise: static, dynamic, ballistic, and proprioceptive neuromuscular facilitation (PNF) (reference). Static and PNF are the most used stretching exercises in fitness and wellness applications. They are safe and effective for improving flexibility. Dynamic and ballistic stretching exercises are commonly used by athletes trained by coaches or athletic trainers. Dynamic and ballistic stretching exercises are not recommended for people whose goals are to improve fitness and wellness as they can pose a greater risk of injuries. Below are the definitions and a specific example for each type of stretching exercise.

Static stretching: Use the range of motion of a joint to stretch muscles slowly and steadily in a held position. For example, we hold our left arm across the body at shoulder level to stretch the left shoulder.

Dynamic stretching: Move a joint repeatedly through a challenging, but comfortable, range of motion necessary for a sport movement. An example of dynamic stretching is swinging legs in a slow, controlled motion.

Ballistic stretching: Move a joint beyond a normal range of motion quickly and briefly by bouncing or rebounding. For example, in a lateral lunge position, perform a ballistic stretch by bouncing up and down.

PNF (proprioceptive neuromuscular facilitation): A muscle is alternatingly stretched passively and contracted. PNF usually requires a partner for assistance. After the initial stretch, body reflexes relax the muscle, and then it can be stretched further. An example of PNF stretching would be if you lay on the floor with one leg straight up in the air, and a partner holds your foot in an upright position. You would apply resistance against your partner's hold to stretch the muscles, and then you would relax them. Your partner then can push on the leg further, and you would apply resistance again to stretch the muscles and then relax them again. This can be repeated several times.

As a teacher or coach, you will educate your students or athletes on the importance and benefits of warming up and cooling down so that they can be properly educated and develop warm-up and cool-down routines. Proper warming up before physical activity can ready the muscles and heart for activities, prevent injuries, and reduce muscle soreness. Proper cooling down after physical activity helps to slow the heart rate gradually and to reduce muscle soreness. Performing stretching exercises helps reduce the risk of injuries and develops and improves flexibility for better fitness and performance.

Background knowledge

For this component, teachers or coaches will need to know the history and culture, rules, and etiquette, needed facilities and equipment, and other resources for sports that they are teaching or coaching.

History and culture

Knowing the history and culture of a sport will help students or athletes to become literate consumers who can appreciate it more. For example, in basketball, teachers or coaches can introduce basketball history and how the sport is connected to American culture. The cultural shift from racial segregation to integration was reflected in basketball games as African Americans were prohibited from playing on White professional teams during the early 1900s and participating in National Basketball Association games prior to 1950. Films such as "Hoosiers", "White Men Can't Jump", "Celtic Pride", "Pistol: The Birth Of A Legend", and "Space Jam" illustrate how basketball has impacted American culture and entertainment, and the role basketball and its superstars play in the daily lives of American households.

Rules and etiquette

Sports are governed by rules. A good understanding of game rules is critical to teaching or coaching sports. There are two different types of rules in sports: primary and secondary rules (Siedentop & van der Mars, 2011). Primary rules define the nature of a sport. They are what make basketball, basketball, rather than football or volleyball, for example, using the hands to dribble, pass, and shoot for points by invading the opponent's court to win a game. Secondary rules are those that can be modified to meet the learners' needs. Examples in basketball include the three-second rule, traveling, number of fouls allowed for each player and team, basket height, ball size, court dimensions, and number of players on a team. For example, when working with seven-year-old-boys on basketball, teachers or coaches can use a junior international size 5 basketball rather than the official adult size. Table 4.1 presents a version of modified basketball rules used with a 3rd and 4th-grade basketball youth league in Dublin Youth Athletics in Ohio.

Sport etiquette refers to a code of expected ethical behaviors from students, athletes, or fans of a particular sport (Martin & Chaney, 2006). It is very important to show etiquette in sports as it demonstrates good sportsperson-ship and respect of other players or fans. For example, good etiquette in sports requires players not to argue with the referees, use bad language, fight with other players, or spit on the floor. All players need to arrive at games on time. Being late is rude and shows bad etiquette. Good etiquette also requires players to greet and shake hands with other players upon arrival or at the end of games. Players who lose the game may even applaud the winning team. However, winners should not applaud themselves by exhibiting their own conceit or pride. Players should not criticize other players, the club, the court, or the surroundings (Martin & Chaney, 2006).

Sport etiquette also applies to fans. For fans, they should respect players, not criticize them, the club, the court, or the surroundings. They should not argue, use bad language, or fight with other fans from opposing teams. They should not throw items at the players or at other fans (Martin & Chaney, 2006) and should not disrupt the game. Learning proper etiquette as well as the game rules is very important for players and spectators to ensure the fairness of games and foster respect and good sportsperson-ship.

Facilities, equipment, and other resources

Teachers or coaches also need to know the facilities and equipment needed for a sport. For example, in basketball, we will need a basketball, goals, and a court to play a game. Whistles, uniforms, scoreboards, computers, etc., are also needed for basketball tournaments. Consulting other resources helps in gaining more knowledge and skill in basketball; such resources include Internet websites, magazines and journals, and books.

Psychomotor skills

To play sports well, an individual must develop competence in various skills. Skill has been "used to describe both the action of controlling the ball and directing the ball, as in ball skills, and the overall effectiveness of the player" (Launder & Piltz, 2013, p.15). In this book, skill is defined as the ability of an individual to perform and/or apply techniques and tactics of a specific sport in a game or non-game context. The term of skill does not include any components of fairness, agility, fitness and endurance, communication, mental toughness, and courage. Those concepts are related to physical conditioning and mental performance, but not associated with techniques and tactics of a sport.

Table 4.1 Modified basketball rules for 3rd and 4th grade youth league

1 Game time is forfeit time. Four players are required to begin the game. Late arrivals on the four-player team may enter the game immediately.
2 Substitutions are permitted at any time for disqualified, injured, or sick players. Otherwise, players must play the entire segment.
3 During overtime and sudden death periods any eligible player may start. Overtime and sudden death periods do not count toward time played.
4 Each team receives two timeouts per half. No carryover of timeouts to the second half or overtime.
5 Three minutes for halftime. Two-minute overtime, continuous clock. Clock stops on whistles during the last 30 seconds of overtime. Sudden death thereafter, with the first team to lead by two points winning. One timeout per team during overtime. No timeouts or substitutions during sudden death.
6 Three-point shots will not be used unless the floor is properly marked.
7 All players must wear the official DYA green and white reversible jersey during games. All numbers are legal.
8 Coaches are permitted one minute for player matchups prior to the start of each quarter.
9 Games will consist of four quarters, a continuous clock, one minute between quarters. Clock stops on whistles during the last two minutes of the second half.
10 All players must play a minimum of one full quarter each half. No player may play more than one quarter more than the teammate who plays the fewest number of quarters.
11 Each third-grade team will have all players present shoot one free throw and one jump shot prior to the start of the game. Each fourth-grade team will have all players present shoot one free throw and one layup (not a jump shot) prior to the start of the game. Each free throw made will count to one point and each jump shot or layup will count one point toward each team's score to start the game. Each player shoots only one free throw and one jump shot or one layup (see league), regardless of the total number of players present for his/her team.
12 Games consist of 8-minute quarters.
13 The free throw line is 9 feet, except 4th grade boys league which is 12 feet. In leagues where the free throw line is 9 feet, the first pair of rebounders must occupy the lane spaces below the block.
14 Zone defenses are prohibited. Man-to-man defense only. Defensive players will pick up the offensive players once they have passed the top of the key extended. If the offense does not penetrate the top of the key extended, the defense can pursue above the top of the key extended. Defensive players must be within 5 feet of their assigned offensive player once the offensive player penetrates the top of the key extended. No trapping outside of the paint. Defense is permitted to double team the ball in the paint area if defensive players are in the paint. Defense may switch to help screened teammates. No backcourt defense or press defense at any time during the game. No four corner of "clear-out" offenses.
15 Lane violation is five seconds.
16 Following time-outs in the last 30 seconds of the game, the clock does not restart until the ball is put into play in the front court.
17 Basket height is 10 feet except third grade girls league which is 9 feet.

Sources: https://dt5602vnjxv0c.cloudfront.net/portals/3789/docs/2023-24%20dya%20basketball%20rules.pdf. Copyrights Obtained.

A sport consists of a variety of skills. Each skill is composed of two components: technique and tactics. Psychomotor skills are composed of two subcomponents, techniques, and tactics, which are defined below. As Launder (2001) argued, psychomotor skill in a sport game is a complex phenomenon. It refers to an effective execution of techniques and tactics in a game. A game's outcome is mainly determined by how skillful the players are in these areas. To win a game, players need to have sound techniques and tactics and be able to execute them effectively and efficiently in a game. At the same time, they need to make good decisions in a game.

Very often, when you watch students or athletes play sports, they make poor decisions and rarely use tactics for offensive or defensive plays. For example, in a soccer game, players all go for the ball, instead of playing for depth, width, and support. As an example, when a teammate is open and there is an open passing lane, a player may fail to apply the two (players) versus one (opponent) tactical play for a better scoring opportunity. When players are not skillful at playing sports and games, it is usually the responsibility of teachers or coaches to teach them the skills. One reason players may not be skillful in a game is that teachers or coaches generally teach them performing techniques soundly rather than psychomotor skills, which is the execution of techniques and tactical plays situated in a game. Another reason is that teachers or coaches may lack knowledge of the psycho-motor skills involved in a sport and how to develop progressive practices to improve their students' or athletes' skills for successful game performances. Therefore, gaining knowledge of the psycho-motor skills involved in a sport and in developing progressive practices is very critical for teachers or coaches to successfully teach or coach that sport.

Techniques

The term "technique" is defined as the way an individual uses their body parts to execute a sport skill. Techniques are the actions that are taken by the player to control and direct the ball in a game (Launder & Piltz, 2013). It consists of all the elements of executing a task. For example, to perform a basketball chest pass, one needs to ensure the presence of various body movement elements in his or her performance, including feet shoulder width apart, back straight, eyes on target, ball held with two hands and palms open, thumbs pointing to each other, ball at chest level, elbows bent up and outward, knees slightly bent, stepping forward to passing direction, shifting weight to the front foot, extending elbows out, releasing the ball off fingers, turning thumbs downward, and following through to passing direction. Those elements are called critical elements since they reflect the sequence of execution of a technique and are critical for technical performance. It is critical for teachers or coaches to know those critical elements for effective teaching or coaching (Chapter 3 presents details on how to develop critical elements of a technique).

A sport has numerous techniques involved in playing the game. For example, in basketball, there are basic movement patterns and footwork, dribbling (speed dribbling, dribbling for close control, post-up dribbling, crossover dribbling, dribbling through the legs, reverse dribbling, spin dribbling, behind-the-back dribbling), shooting (bank shot, jump shot, hook shot, lay-up, reverse lay-up, fade-away jump shot, free throw), catching, passing (bounce, overhead, chest pass, one-handed pass), rebounding/boxing out, shot blocking, triple threat positioning, and cutting and screening. Teachers or coaches should have an in-depth knowledge of those techniques and which techniques for which age groups and skill levels for effective teaching or coaching.

Tactics

Tactic is defined as decision-making, strategies, and offensive and defensive movements relative to the rules of a sport that are carefully planned by a player or players to win a game (Launder, 2001). Tactics have two different types: offensive and defensive. An example of an offensive tactic in basketball is that after passing the ball to his or her teammate, an offensive player needs to move to an open space to support his or her teammates. Other basketball offensive tactics include fast break, pick and roll, support, ball possession, faking, give and go, 1-on-1, 2-on-1, 3-on-1, and 3-on-2, etc. An example of a defensive tactic in basketball is that a defensive player moves to double team an offensive player with the ball to support his teammate. Other defensive tactics include zone defense (2-1-2, 2-3, 1-2-2) and man-to-man defense.

Not only do teachers need to have knowledge in those techniques and tactics, but also shall know what techniques and tactics to teach for students at different developmental stages (Li et al., 2018). For example, this point of view also applied to coaching at what age group should a physical education teacher introduce the technique of dribbling with a full turn 180 degree or individual fake-deception tactics in a soccer unit? In a study by Li et al. (2018), the authors mapped out soccer techniques and tactics that should be taught to 9- to 14-year-old students in physical education. The findings demonstrate that certain soccer techniques and tactics can only be taught to students at certain age levels. A knowledge of these age-developmentally appropriate techniques and tactics can provide critical guidance for teachers or coaches to plan their teaching or coaching progressively, thus improving their instruction quality and maximizing students' or athletes' learning and performance.

Progressive practices

In addition to identifying the techniques and tactics, another aspect of a macro sports analysis is to possess the knowledge of progressive practices that can be used to advance students' or athletes' learning and performance from the current level to next level. Progressive practices are tasks/activities/concepts sequenced in a manner that moves students from the less complex and sophisticated to more difficult and complicated tasks by adding complexity. Many factors have an impact on task complexity, including the space and boundaries of the play area, equipment, number of players, game rules, game conditions, tactics and problems, attacker/defender ratio, nature of the goal, and nature of the skills (closed versus open) (Chapter 5 will discuss how these factors affect the task complexity in detail).

For example, one way to increase the difficulty level is to modify a closed skill to an open skill. A closed skill is a skill performed in a fixed environment, where the performance conditions remain constant. An open skill is a skill performed in an ever-changing environment, where the performance conditions are variable. For a closed skill, teachers or coaches will mainly focus on refining the critical technical elements that are performed invariably. For an open skill, teachers or coaches will spend less time on technical elements and more time on extending tasks that cover the variety of situations where the skill will be applied in games. Using basketball shooting as an example, teachers or coaches can start with a stationary foul shot. This is a closed skill where the emphasis will be the technical elements of executing shooting and the practice condition remains constant. To increase the difficulty and complexity, teachers or coaches can have students practice shooting with a passive defender, who will put up the arms with the intent to block the shot. This is an open skill where the emphasis will be on how to respond to the movement of the defender and the practice condition is variable.

As stated earlier, progressive practices are designed from less complex and difficult to more complex and difficult tasks that are more situated in a real-life game. By changing or combining characteristics of tasks in a skill, numerous progressions can be developed for skill development. Progressive practices have a snowball-like effect, always increasing in size by adding different layers. Table 4.2 presents a soccer dribbling for close control progression. The first progression is dribbling for close control with a back-away defender from the baseline to the midline. Having a defender ensures that the task presents a game-like scenario, and that the offensive player keeps his eyes up rather than looking at the ball, which is a common mistake students or players make. In the second and third progressions, having a defender step into the dribbling direction forces the offensive player to use cuts (inside, progression 2, or outside, progression 3) to change direction, which increases the difficulty. By adding turns and multiple defenders while allowing no stealing, progression 4 becomes more difficult, with more game-like elements. In progression 5, defenders are allowed to steal the ball. For progressions 6–8, dribbling techniques become more difficult with various degrees of defense, which enables students and players to become more skillful. By adding other soccer skills such as passing and shooting, the rest of the progressions become more complex as more skills are involved. The progressive practices can get "bigger and bigger" by changing game parameters related to dribbling and passing as other skills are added. These progressive practices can move students or athletes successfully from one level to the next. Students or athletes

Table 4.2 Progressive practices for soccer dribbling for close control

1 Dribble for close control with a back-away defender from one baseline to the midline
2 Dribble for close control with a defender stepping into the dribbling direction to force the dribbler to change direction using inside cut from one baseline to the midline
3 Dribble for close control with a defender stepping into the dribbling direction to force the dribbler to change direction using outside cut from one baseline to the midline
4 Dribble for close control using cuts and turns in a circle with defenders (no stealing)
5 Dribble for close control using cuts and turns in a circle with defenders actively stealing the ball
6 Use right foot roll across the ball and use left foot in-step to cut and get past a stationary defender
7 Use right foot roll across the ball and left foot in-step to cut and get past a warm defender
8 Use right foot roll across the ball and left foot in-step to cut and get past an active defender
9 Receive a pass and then use right foot roll across the ball and left foot in-step to cut and get past a stationary defender
10 Receive a pass and then use right foot roll across the ball and left foot in-step to cut and get pasts a warm defender
11 Receive a pass and then use right foot roll across the ball and left foot in-step to cut and get past an active defender
12 Use right foot roll across the ball and use left foot in-step to cut and get past a stationary defender, and then shoot for a goal
13 Use right foot roll across the ball and use left foot in-step to cut and get past a warm defender, and then shoot for a goal
14 Use right foot roll across the ball and use left foot in-step to cut and get past an active defender, and then shoot for a goal
15 Receive a pass, use right foot roll across the ball and use left foot in-step to cut and get past a stationary defender, and then shoot for a goal
16 Receive a pass, use right foot roll across the ball and use left foot in-step to cut and get past a warm defender, and then shoot for a goal
17 Receive a pass, use right foot roll across the ball and use left foot in-step to cut and get past an active defender, and then shoot for a goal

can also easily apply them in games as these practices should be designed based on the scenarios taken from real games. Using a similar approach, Table 4.3 presents an example progressive practice for a basketball chest pass in Table 4.2. Due to space considerations, only partial progressive practices are listed in Tables 4.2 and 4.3. Chapter 5 will present a fuller discussion on how to design progressive practices, also called task progressions.

Psycho-social concepts

To be successful at playing sports, individuals need to have a good understanding of the game rules, use effective skills and tactics, and be in good

Table 4.3 Progressive practices for basketball chest pass

1 Make a stationary pass and move to an open space: In a square with three players on three corners, pass a ball to one of the other two players and move to the open corner

2 Move and pass from middle line to baseline: Two players pass the ball back and forth while moving from midline to baseline

3 Make a stationary pass and move to an open space with a cold defender: In a square with three players on three corners, pass a ball to one of the other two players and move to the open corner. The defender will position in front of the ball player with hands up (no stealing)

4 Make a stationary pass and move to an open space with a warm defender: In a square with three players on three corners, pass a ball to one of the other two players and move to the open corner. The defender will move to block passing lane with hands moving up and down (no stealing)

5 Make a stationary pass and move to an open space with an active defender: In a square with three players on three corners, pass a ball to one of the other two players and move to the open corner. The defender will actively defend and try to steal the ball.

6 Move and pass from midline to baseline with a cold defender: Two players pass the ball back and forth while moving from midline to baseline. The defender positions his or her body close to the ball player and move back in the middle with no stealing

7 Move and pass from midline to baseline with a warm defender: Two players pass the ball back and forth while moving from midline to baseline. The defender positions his or her body close to the ball player and apply pressure but with no stealing

8 Move and pass from midline to baseline with an active defender: Two players pass the ball back and forth while moving from midline to baseline. The defender will defend the ball player actively with stealing.

9 2 versus 0: The ball player passes the ball to the other player, cuts to basket, receives the pass from the other player, and then shoots the basket (layup or jump shot).

10 2 versus 1: The ball player passes the ball to the other player, cuts to basket, receives the pass from the other player, and then shoots the basket (layup or jump shot). The defense will assume a stationary position to defend the ball player with hands up.

11 2 versus 1: The ball player passes the ball to the other player, cuts to basket, receives the pass from the other player, and then shoots the basket (layup or jump shot). The defense will assume a position to defend the ball player with warm defense by moving feet and hands (no stealing).

12 2 versus 1: The ball player passes the ball to the other player, cuts to basket, receives the pass from the other player, and then shoots the basket (layup or jump shot). The defense will actively defend the ball player with stealing.

physical condition. In addition, students or athletes will need to possess critical psycho-social attributes that contribute to success in sports: such as (1) being a team player; (2) having self-confidence, perseverance, discipline, drive, and self-management skills; and (3) assuming personal and social responsibility. Many real-world examples demonstrate the importance of players working together to win games in team sports. No matter whether we play a pick-up, league, or professional game, one or two players cannot win it all by themselves. Winning games requires the efforts of the entire team with every player on the court or field contributing to winning a championship. Self-confidence, perseverance, discipline, drive, responsibility, and self-management skills are all critical for a person to be successful in sports, and in their daily lives as well.

When teaching or coaching a sport, teachers or coaches must be aware of these key psycho-social attributes and purposely instill them in their students or athletes. To enhance a player's self-confidence and perseverance, teachers or coaches can emphasize the efficacy of effort, foster a task mastery and individual improvement learning environment, teach SMART goal setting (Table 4.4) (Doran, 1981; Locke, & Latham, 2013, 2015), focus students or athletes on playing sports for enjoyment and fun, and create a successful playing experience. An example of a SMART goal is "In order to get in better shape, I will run 3 miles at least 5 times a week. By the end of 12 weeks, my goal is to run the 3 miles in 28 minutes".

To systematically foster discipline, responsibility, and self-management skills, teachers or coaches can use curricular/instructional models to teach or coach sports, which focus on character development. Those curricular/instructional models include Sport Education (Siedentop, 1994; Siedentop et al., 2011), Adventure-based Learning (Bisson, 1999; Cosgriff, 2000; Frank, 2004), Teaching Personal and Social Responsibility (Hellison, 2011), and Cooperative Learning (Dyson & Casey, 2012). Or teachers or coaches can use some of the instructional strategies from these curricular/instructional models to empower students or athletes with choices, responsibilities, and opportunities for self-management and leadership.

Numerous adventure-based and cooperative games and activities can also be used to develop teamwork, leadership, discipline, personal and social responsibility, self-challenging, communication, resilience, self-control, and self-management skills (Rohnke, 2009). For example, the magic stick game can be used to develop teamwork, self-control, respect, and communication skills. The objective of the magic stick game is to lower a stick (a long stick or

Table 4.4 SMART goals

SMART	Definition
"S" for "specific"	A goal is specific when it states exactly what we want to happen, what we are going to do, why it is important to us, and how we are going to do it.
"M" for "measurable"	A goal is measurable when our progress toward achieving it can be seen and measured.
"A" for "attainable".	A goal is attainable when it is within our reach.
"R" for "realistic".	A realistic goal is one that is doable for us.
"T" for "timely".	A goal is timely when it specifies a timeframe for achieving it.

tent pole) to the ground while all participating students or athletes keep their fingers straight and touch the stick. Students or athletes make two lines facing each other. Each student or athlete puts both pointer fingers out straight at chest level. Students or athletes facing each other should have their fingers set "every other" with those across from them. The Magic Stick is set along the group's fingers. Students or athletes must lower the stick to the ground while keeping their fingers straight and always touching the stick. The stick should be reset if students curl their fingers around the stick, make an X with their fingers, or use other fingers to lower the stick. Very often, students or athletes will get frustrated and scream at one another. A few students or athletes will dominate the activity. Students or athletes can recognize the importance of teamwork, self-control, respect, and communication through guided group debriefs after a couple trials, and then develop those characteristics by repeatedly doing this until they can successfully complete the game.

For another example, leadership can be fostered by empowering students or athletes with different roles such as team captain, equipment manager, or leader for warm-up, cool-down, or stretching exercises, etc. Cooperation or teamwork can be developed by using a good behavioral point system to hold students or athletes accountable at the team level. The following is an example of a good behavior point system: All teams start with zero points. Teams will earn points in each of the three behavioral categories listed below. A maximum of 9 points can be given per day. Teachers or coaches can also award additional bonus points for exceptional behaviors and significant improvement. The good behavior point system has been very effective in building good sportsperson-ship and character among students or athletes.

i Be a team player and follow assigned roles (3 points)
ii Be a good sport by respecting players, teachers or coaches, and equipment (3 points)
iii Help and care for other teammates (3 points)

How to conduct sports analysis

Conducting sports analysis seems to be an overwhelming task. However, it will become easier if teachers or coaches follow the steps described in this section. The sequence for steps 2 to 6 is not locked in. Teachers or coaches can work on these steps in any order and then put them all together before they move on to do step 7. Upon the completion of sports analysis, teachers or coaches will produce a knowledge package where they establish a database for their teaching or coaching. In the future, teachers or coaches can pick and choose the content to develop their unit and lesson plans or coaching practices based on the developmental levels of their students or athletes. The "knowledge package" has all the seasonings and foods such as meats, seafood, and veggies, etc. Just like a cooking chef, he or she prepares the meals based on the likes of his or her customers.

Step 1: Collect information

The first step is to gather all the information related to the sport(s) that teachers or coaches will teach or coach. The information can be history, techniques, tactics, game rules, facilities, practices, etc. Many resources are available from which teachers or coaches can find the information, such as books, websites, journals in coaching or physical education, or coaches/university professors in the field. Teachers or coaches can borrow some books from the library or purchase them if they have the financial resources. Teachers or coaches can search the Internet for the sport, but keep in mind that teachers or coaches will need to be critical about what they find to distinguish good content from bad. Do not use the information from just any website. We recommend three criteria for teachers or coaches to judge the quality of content on a website: First, teachers or coaches should check the credibility of the organization hosting the site that provides the online materials. Has the organization been accredited by national associations? If it is accredited, very often teachers or coaches can trust the quality of content provided. Second, teachers or coaches should check the credentials of the authors of the material on the site. Do they have any certificates or degrees in sport coaching or teaching? What kind of sport experience do they have? What kind of teaching or coaching background do the authors have? In general, authors with a certificate or degree in sports coaching or teaching, a lot of experience in playing sports at competitive levels, and a lot of coaching or teaching experience would provide more trustworthy, higher quality content than those without such a background. Lastly, teachers or coaches should check the quality of the content itself. If the online material provides instructions, are they clear and detailed? Do any steps seem to be missing? Do they provide any demonstrations in the form of drawings, photos, or videos? Do the authors provide a series of progressive practices for skill development? Online materials that include such information are of better quality and more trustworthy than those who do not. After you have gathered all the information, the next step for teachers or coaches is to organize and synthesize it for their teaching or coaching preparations.

Step 2: Develop a database of history and culture of sports for teaching or coaching

In this step, teachers or coaches will review the information about the history and culture of sports they have collected and develop a database of the history and culture of sports for their teaching or coaching. Using basketball as an example, teachers or coaches can discuss when and where James Naismith invented basketball, how basketball games have evolved since 1891, and how the game has influenced American culture and the daily lives of American households. Teachers or coaches can also use movies to demonstrate the cultural shift from racial segregation to integration.

Step 3: Build a database of warm-up, cool-down, and stretching exercises

As we discussed earlier, it is very important for students or players to warm-up before playing sports and cool-down after playing sports. Doing stretching exercises before and after will also help prevent injury and develop flexibility for better performance and fitness. In step 3, teachers or coaches should build a database of numerous warm-up, cool-down, and stretching exercises for them to use in their future teaching or coaching. Using soccer as an example, students or athletes can jog a couple laps to warm up and then stretch their arms, necks, shoulders, back, legs, knees, and ankles, using static and dynamic stretches. After the general warm-up and stretching exercises, students or athletes can juggle, head, dribble, pass, and shoot a ball as sports-specific warm-up exercises. After playing soccer, students or athletes can cool down by walking for a couple laps to allow their heart to slow down gradually and then do more general stretching exercises to develop flexibility.

Step 4: Build a database for physical training workouts for different age groups

Physical conditioning is critical not only for injury prevention but also successful performance in sports. For example, to achieve optimal performance in basketball and soccer, players need to have excellent cardiovascular capacity, muscular strength and endurance, and flexibility. As a teacher or youth coach, you can adopt physical training workouts from your peers or other experts in this area. You will also need to develop the competency to design physical training workouts for your students or youth athletes to improve their physical condition. Those physical training workouts must be developmentally appropriate since children's and youth's physical, cognitive, emotional, and social skills are at different developmental levels for different age groups. In this chapter, we will provide an overview but not discuss how to develop a physical training workout in detail as there are many published books on this topic.

To develop a physical training workout, teachers or coaches must know the FITT formula (Frequency, Intensity, Time, and Type; see Table 4.5 for definitions) and the basic training principles (Corbin & Lindsey, 2006; Siedentop & van der Mars, 2011). The basic training principles include progressive overload, specificity, reversibility, recovery time, and individuality (Corbin & Lindsey, 2006; Siedentop & van der Mars, 2011).

Table 4.5 The FITT formula

Term	Definitions
Frequency	How many times should a person exercise a week?
Intensity	How hard should a person exercise?
Time	How long should a person exercise during each session?
Type	What types of exercises should a person perform?

Specificity: Training should be directly related to intended performance. In other words, the selection of exercises must specifically match our conditioning goals. For example, if the goal is to improve aerobic capacity, one must run or swim rather than do push-ups or sit-ups.

Progressive overload: Do more than what the body can do gradually. For example, to improve muscular strength, one will have to do more than what his or her muscles can normally do. The exercise loads must be increased gradually. Doing too much or increasing exercise loads significantly in a short period of time can lead to injuries.

Recovery time: After exercising, allow the body time for rest and repair. If the body does not get time for rest and repair, this can lead to overuse of body muscles, joints, ligaments, and tendons. Over time, overuse can lead to some injuries.

Reversibility: If you do not use it, you will lose it. The functions of your body muscles and organs will decrease if you do not exercise to maintain or improve them. If you regularly lift weights twice a week, your muscles will lose strength and endurance if you do not lift for several weeks.

Individuality: Individuals have different personalities, physical ability, and skills. Therefore, a training program needs to consider different exercise preferences as well as different responses to training. When designing exercise workouts, teachers or coaches will need to select exercises and loads based on their students' or players' interests and what they can accomplish. Teachers or coaches should also emphasize to students and players that their bodies may respond to training differently than the bodies of their peers, so they should concentrate on their own workout and focus on personal improvement rather than comparing themselves to others. If students or athletes focus on comparing themselves with others, they may put themselves at risk for injuries.

As discussed above, one goal of a physical conditioning program should be to improve flexibility. Recall that the goal of doing stretching is to develop flexibility of the muscles, joints, tendons, and ligaments. By applying the FITT formula and basic training principles to stretching, a flexibility training program could specify that individuals perform stretching exercises before and after each exercise session 7 days a week. Each stretch should be performed at least twice and should be held for 10–15 seconds each. The stretches should produce slight muscular discomfort and progress from minimal applied resistance to more applied resistance to increase flexibility. As training continues, students or athletes can gradually increase the number of stretches and the amount of applied resistance using the progressive overload principle.

The second goal of a physical conditioning program is to increase muscle strength and endurance, and weightlifting is often used to increase both. Muscular strength is defined as the maximal force that those muscles can produce against a resistance. One repetition maximum (1 rm) is commonly used to measure muscular strength. You can obtain our 1RM by performing an exercise using a safe weight for 6–12 repetitions, then using this formula to calculate 1RM= ((The number of repetitions x 0.3) + 1) x the original amount of weight lifted. Muscular endurance refers to the ability of muscles to exert force against a resistance over a period. Partial curl-up and push-up tests are normally recommended for measuring endurance of the abdominal muscles and the upper body, respectively.

A weight training program should consist of a program goal, the amount of resistance per lift, number of repetitions per set, number of sets per workout, and number of workouts per week. Teachers and coaches use the program goals and students' or players' training status to determine these specifications. Using the FITT formula, a weight training program for beginners might specify that they perform weightlifting 2–3 times per week with an intensity of 60–70% of one maximum repetition, and 10–15 repetitions per set with a rest of 1–2 minutes between sets. For general conditioning, individuals can perform weightlifting 2–3 times per week with an intensity of 60–80% of one maximum repetition, and 8–12 repetitions per set with a rest of 2–3 minutes between sets. For advanced training, individuals can perform weightlifting 4–6 times per week with an intensity of 70–100% of one maximum repetition, and 1–12 repetitions per set. At this level, there is a rest of at least three minutes between sets (Hopson, Donatelle, & Littrell, 2012). The number of sets per workout can range from 2–5. After a period of training, muscles adapt to the training. Then students or athletes should apply the progressive overload principle to continue to increase muscular strength and endurance by increasing the amount of resistance per lift, the number of repetitions per set, or the number of sets per workout.

A third goal of a physical conditioning program is to develop cardio-vascular capacity, and conditioning programs frequently use running, jogging, playing certain sports, and doing certain fitness activities to achieve this goal. Cardio-vascular capacity is defined as the ability of the heart, lungs, and organs to supply oxygen to body muscles and tissues and the ability to adjust to and recover from sustained physical activity. Applying the FITT formula, a conditioning program to increase cardio-vascular capacity among beginners might specify that they exercise at least 30 minutes three times per week with an intensity of 50–69% maximum heart rate (the highest heart rate attainable during exercise, usually estimated with the formula: maximum HR = 220 − age). For intermediate students or players, they should exercise 40–60 minutes 3–5 times per week with an intensity of 60–75% maximum heart rate. For advanced students or players, they should exercise 60–120 minutes 5–6 times per week with an intensity of 65–90% maximum heart rate (reference).

Step 5: Build a database of game rules for different age groups

Game rules must be developmentally appropriate for the age of the learners. To teach or coach basketball, for example, to children and youth, the official NBA or college basketball game rules must be modified to be developmentally appropriate for them. Very often, teachers or coaches do not need to develop the game rules from scratch for children and youth as numerous youth leagues in the community have probably already done an excellent job of modifying the regular adult game rules to be developmentally appropriate for children. For example, in Ohio, Dublin Youth Athletics has developed different basketball rules for different grade levels (1st and 2nd grade boys' and girls' leagues; 3rd and 4th grade boys' and girls' leagues, see Table 4.1; 5th and 6th grade boys' and girls' leagues; and 7th–12th boys' and girls' leagues). Teachers or coaches can just adopt them or make some adaptations for the children and youth that they teach or coach.

Step 6: Develop a database of skills and progressive practices

Teachers or coaches must possess knowledge of techniques, tactics, and progressive practices to effectively teach or coach a sport. An effective teacher or coach must know these techniques, tactics, and progressive practices like the back of his or her hand. This is the most important step in conducting sport analysis. The process of developing a database of skills and progressive practices is time consuming. However, it is worthwhile and rewarding as it provides a foundation for effective teaching or coaching. First, teachers or coaches will need to identify and categorize all the psycho-motor skills (techniques and tactics) related to the sport that they will teach or coach. Since teachers to coaches have collected resources with this information in step 1, here they will group the skills into different categories based on the types of techniques and tactics. Then, teachers or coaches will need to develop a series of progressive practices designed to improve these psycho-motor skills so that their students or athletes can succeed in games. In Chapter 8, we will fully discuss how to develop progressive practices/task progressions. Figure 4.1 provides a template that can be used to guide you in conducting an analysis of psycho-motor skills. By following this template, teachers or coaches will experience less frustration during the process of conducting an analysis of psycho-motor skills.

Step 7: Map out skills and progressive practices for students or athletes with different skill levels

Students or athletes come to play sports with varying skills and ability sets and grow at a different rate. When teachers or coaches teach or coach a sport to children and youth, they must be able to know which skills and progressive practices are more developmentally appropriate based on their ability and skill levels so that they can improve and succeed. From step 6, teachers or coaches have developed a database of all the techniques, tactics, and progressive practices that they need to teach or coach a sport. Now in step 7, teachers or coaches will need to map out the skills and progressive practices for the specific ages or levels of students or athletes. The skills and progressive practices that teachers or coaches use for 11-year-old children are different from those for youth at age 15 years. Even for the same age group of children and youth, they will have different skill sets, characteristics, and interests, and

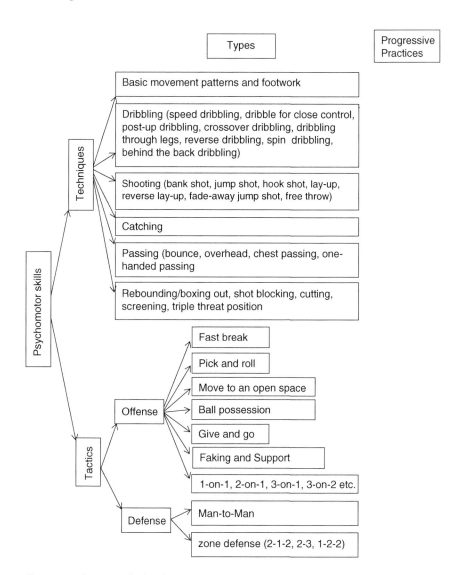

Figure 4.1 Sport analysis of psycho-motor skills for basketball.

will learn and grow at a different rate. If the tasks are too easy, they will not help students or athletes successfully move up to the next level. If the tasks are too difficult, students or athletes will very often not have successful experiences. Unsuccessful experiences usually have a negative impact on students' or players' emotions, which can eventually produce a negative impact on their performance.

Therefore, it is a very important skill for teachers or coaches to define and sequence the content to be taught to different age groups. A sport consists of a variety of techniques and tactics. Which technique(s) or tactics should be taught to a specific age group? In the article by Li et al. (2018), the authors took the first step to map out what soccer techniques and tactics should be taught to 3rd–8th graders in physical education. This article provides some guidance for teachers or coaches to map out developmentally appropriate skills for different age groups. Table 4.6 presents a template for mapping out basketball techniques and tactics for different age groups. The first column consists of major footwork, techniques, and tactics. The second column contains specific types of footwork, techniques, and tactics. The third column is age groups with subcategories of 3rd to 6th grades. Teachers or coaches can check a box if a specific footwork, technique, or tactic is appropriately taught to a specific grade. You can also read the article by Li et al. (2018) to see the soccer example.

Content maps can be used to map out progressive practices, which is a graphic representation of content development/progression (Ward et al., 2017). It displays a hierarchical structure of intratask development from an initial and easy task to more complex tasks and the relationship of intertask development when two different types of tasks are combined. Intratask means within a task. Intertask means between tasks. For example, stationary passing in partners is an intratask of passing while moving in partners. Stationary passing in partners is an intertask of stationary shooting two feet away from the basket. Content map provides a tool for teachers or coaches to define and select appropriate content to be taught for different age groups (Ward et al., 2017; Ward et al., 2015).

To create a content map, teachers or coaches can start with the basic content areas to be taught in terms of skills and tactics with a short description of the task and then list them vertically in the sequence from an initial and easy task to more complex tasks using an arrow. Finally, teachers or coaches diagram the relationships among the intertasks using an angled arrow (Ward et al., 2017; Ward et al., 2015). Please see Figure 4.2 for an example of a basketball content map. Teachers or coaches can also develop a content map for a specific grade group. More examples are provided in the article by Ward et al. (2015).

Step 8: Build a database of games and activities for developing psycho-social concepts

There are numerous psycho-social concepts that teachers or coaches can instill during their teaching or coaching, including hard work, teamwork, self-challenge, self-management, self-discipline, self-confidence, problem solving, learning community, self-motivation, etc. All those psycho-social concepts can be fostered through adventurous and cooperative games and activities. Based on the types of sports one teaches or coaches, he or she will need to determine the specific psycho-social attributes to emphasize and what effective strategies can be used to develop them successfully.

Table 4.6 Mapping out age-appropriate techniques and tactics

Categories of techniques and tactics	Content	Frequency used in games			
		Third grade	Fourth grade	Fifth grade	Sixth grade
Basic Stances and Movements	Basic stance (Preparation, triple-threat, defense)				
	Faking movement				
	Change of pace/direction				
	V-cut				
	Inside/outside cut				
	Turn and run				
	Sideward running				
	Back pedal				
	Slide/shuffle				
Dribbling	Stationary dribble				
	Drive/ break				
	Change-of-pace dribbling				
	Crossover dribbling on the move				
	Spin dribbling on the move				
	Between-legs dribbling on the move				
	Behind-the-back dribbling on the move				

Passing and Catching	Both hands chest pass				
	Single hand chest pass				
	Side-arm pass				
	Side bounce pass				
	Both hands overhand pass				
	Baseball pass				
	Behind the back pass				
	Between-legs pass				
	Long pass				
Shooting	Free throw				
	Three-point shot				
	Underhand layup				
	Overhand layup				
	Reverse layup/lay in				
	Hook shot				
	Jump shot				
	Floater shot				
	Dunk/slam				

(*Continued*)

Table 4.6 (Continued)

Categories of techniques and tactics	Content	Frequency used in games			
		Third grade	*Fourth grade*	*Fifth grade*	*Sixth grade*
	Tip shot				
Rebounding	Stationary rebound				
	Crash the board				
	Box out				
Jump ball	Jump ball				
Offensive Tactics	Give and go				
	Screen				
	Drive and pass				
	Support				
	Pick and roll				
	Fast break				
	1v0				
	1v1				
	2v1				
	2v2				

3v2					
3v3					
4v3					
4v4					
5v4					
5v5					
1v2					
2v3					
3v4					
4v5					
Defensive Tactics	Switch				
	Push through				
	Pressure				
	Close				
	1v1				
	2v1				
	2v2				
	3v2				

(Continued)

Table 4.6 (Continued)

Categories of techniques and tactics	Content	Frequency used in games			
		Third grade	Fourth grade	Fifth grade	Sixth grade
	3v3				
	4v3				
	4v4				
	5v4				
	5v5				
	1v2				
	2v3				
	3v4				
	4v5				
	Zone defense				
	Man to man defense				

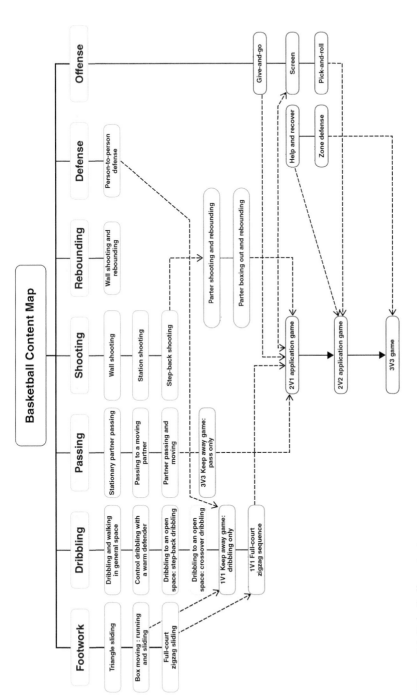

Figure 4.2 Basketball content map.

Summary

In this chapter, we have discussed the definitions of sports analysis, technique, skill, tactics, and progressive practices. It is very important for teachers or coaches to distinguish the differences between technique, skill, and tactics. Sports analysis is composed of four components (physiological training and conditioning, background knowledge, psychomotor skills (techniques, tactics, and progressive practices) and there are eight steps that teachers or coaches can follow to successfully conduct sports analysis. After completing this chapter, teachers or coaches should be able to conduct sports analysis of a sport with which they teach or coach.

Questions for reflection

- What is sports analysis? What are the purposes of conducting sports analysis?
- What is the definition of technique, skill, and tactics?
- How are technique, skill, and tactic similar to or different from each other?
- What are the five components of sports analysis?
- What are the eight steps to conduct sports analysis?

References

Bisson, C. (1999). Sequencing the adventure experience. In J. Miles & S. Priest (Eds.), *Adventure programming* (pp. 205–214). State College, PA: Venture Publishing.

Corbin, C. B., & Lindsey, R. (2006). *Fitness for life* (5th ed.). Champion, IL: Human Kinetics.

Cosgriff, M. (2000). Walking our talk: Adventure based learning and physical education. *Journal of Physical Education New Zealand, 33,* 89–98.

Doran, G. T. (1981). There's a S.M.A.R.T. way to write management's goals and objectives. *Management Review, 70,* 35–36.

Dyson, B., & Casey, A. (2012). *Cooperative learning in physical education: A research-based approach.* London: Routledge.

Frank, L. S. (2004). *Journey toward the caring classroom: Using adventure to create community.* Oklahoma City, OK: Woods 'N' Barnes Publishing & Distribution.

Hellison, D. (2011). *Teaching responsibility through physical activity* (3rd ed.). Champaign, IL: Human Kinetics.

Hopson, J. L., Donatelle, R. J., & Littrell, T. R. (2012). *Get fit, stay well.* (2nd ed.). San Francisco, CA: Benjamin Cummings.

Launder, A. (2001). *Play practice: The games approach to teaching and coaching sports.* Champion, IL: Human Kinetics.

Launder, A., & Piltz, W. (2013). *Play practice.* Champion, IL: Human Kinetics.

Li, W., Dervent, F., & Xie, X. (2018). Soccer techniques and tactics for third- through eighth-grade students in physical education. *Journal of Physical Education, Recreation & Dance, 89*(8), 23–28.

Locke, E. A., & Latham, G. P. (2013). *New developments in goal setting and task performance.* Routledge.

Locke, E. A., & Latham, G. P. (2015). Breaking the rules: A historical overview of goal-setting theory. In A. J. Elliot (Ed.), *Advances in motivation science* (Vol. 2, pp. 99–126). Elsevier

Martin, J. S., & Chaney, L. H. (2006). *Global business etiquette: A guide to international communication and customs*. Westport, CT: Praeger Publishers.

Rohnke, K. (2009). *Silver bullets: A revised guide to initiative problems, adventure games, and trust activities*. Dubuque, IA: Kendall Hunt Publishing.

Siedentop, D. (1994). *Sport Education: Quality PE through positive sport experiences*. Champaign, IL: Human Kinetics.

Siedentop, D., Hastie, P., & van der Mars, H. (2011). *Complete guide to sport education*. Champaign, IL: Human Kinetics.

Siedentop, D., & van der Mars, H. (2011). *Introduction to physical education, fitness, and sport* (8th ed.). New York, NY: McGraw Hill.

Ward, P., Lee, Y. S., Kim, I., Dervent, F., Ko, B., & Tao, W. (2017). Using content maps to measure content development in physical education: Validation and application. *Journal of Teaching in Physical Education, 36*, 20–31.

Ward, P., Lehwald, H., & Lee, Y. S. (2015). Content maps: A teaching and assessment tool for content knowledge. *Journal of Physical Education, Health. Recreation and Dance, 86*(5), 46–54. 10.1080/07303084.2015.1022675.

5   Understanding movement preparation

Outcomes

- Understand the differential definitions of perception between Information Processing Theory and Ecological Approach.
- Utilize the measure of reaction time to quantify movement preparation.
- Identify the factors that will influence movement preparation.
- Understand the role of attention in preparation for successful movements.

The skillful movements are often well-planned before execution, either with or without consciousness of the performer. Therefore, the first step for skill analysis is to examine what information is used by a performer to prepare and plan for the required movements, and what factors could have influenced the utilization of such information. These questions are shared by cognitive scientists who have studied perception and attention for centuries, and their empirical findings have been informative and suggestive for movement scientists and practitioners.

Perception and movement preparation

What precedes the production of a skillful movement? "To be is to be perceived", a quote from George Berkeley, a philosopher in 18th century, who has suggested that nothing exists outside of our perception (Downing, 2004). In other words, one can sense the stimulation from the surroundings through our powerful sensory system (i.e., seeing, hearing, touching), but one can never interpret this sensory information without perception. Therefore, perception is a process by which meaning is attached to sensory information. Then, a natural question to follow is: where is the meaning coming from? Two theoretical models have been proposed to account for perception, in which the origin of the "meaning" is stipulated from different perspectives.

Perception understood in information processing theory

As a guiding theory for cognitive science, the information processing (IP) theory (Simon, 1978) is known for its three stages of processing that are supposed to happen between input (stimulus) and output (motor response):

DOI: 10.4324/9781003331964-7

stimulus detection, stimulus identification, and response selection. Supposing a man is walking in the park and there is a flying ball coming at him: First, he has to detect whether there is a ball coming his way; then he has to identify the characteristics of the ball including its size, shape, and flying features (e.g., speed, trajectory, or spin); finally, he has to select an appropriate action in response to the flying ball (e.g., dodging or catching with one or two hands). Apparently, perception is required and involved in all stages of information processing, and it even facilitates the transition from one stage to another. However, how could the "meaning" be attached to enable the staged processing? According to the IP theory, the memory system is also involved in the staged processing. The system-registered stimulus will be encoded, stored, and retrieved to become meaningful. In other words, if the stimulus is something similar to what has been experienced or learned previously, it will be more meaningful, therefore, easier for detection, identification, and then selection for response.

Based on the IP theory, perception is a cognitive process that must happen and complete before any overt action can be generated, and the mistakes seen in executing a motor skill must be attributed to the misperception of the task and environment relevant to the motor skill. Consequently, to minimize the action errors, one must train the perceptual system to be alert and only responsive to the skill-relevant stimuli while ignoring the skill-irrelevant stimuli. For instance, a skilled soccer goalkeeper must attend to the following perceptual information before a successful action of stopping a goal can be generated:

• The foot used to kick the ball
• Ball characteristics including velocity, trajectory, spin, and direction
• The score
• The sight and sound of the crowd
• The smell and color of the grass
• The feel of sweat on skin

Since the superior action is merely a result of superior perception according to the IP theory, the perceptual training focused on learning the perceptual information relevant to goalkeeping is deemed as more important than physical practice of goalkeeping in developing the motor skill of goalkeeping.

Perception understood in ecological approach

The ecological approach (EA) differs from the IP theory in that it gives equal importance to perception and action. The EA embraces the dynamical systems approach to skill acquisition (Vereijken et al., 1992), considering that skilled movements are functional as they are the optimal solutions for the performer to solve the problems encountered in the ever-changing situation. Since the situation keeps changing, the perceptual system needs to capture the changes to inform the action system to change as well. Meanwhile, the consequence of the action is causing situational changes, therefore, must be perceived to inform the decision of whether keeping or changing the action. Such a circular relationship between perception and action is maintained until the situational problem is solved.

Three factors are known to interact to support the circular relationship between perception and action: environment, task, and individual. The environmental factors include external objects, conditions, and people that could have impacted both perception and action of an individual in performing the motor skill. The task factors include equipment, time, instructions, goals, and rules that an individual must use and follow in performing the motor skill. The individual factors include cognitive and motor abilities, previous experience, and motivation that could have limited or enabled an individual to perform the motor skill. Nonetheless, each of these three factors is ever-changing and they are also interacting with one another to determine what is perceived and how to act.

The concept of "affordances" is often used to capture such a triangular relationship that determines both perception and action subserving a motor skill. According to Gibson (1977), affordances are action possibilities that emerge by relating the environmental and/or task factors with the individual factor. For instance, to receive a thrown ball, one can use one hand or two hands depending on the ball size in relation to one's own hand size. For a fixed hand size, a large ball (e.g., basketball) will be caught with two hands while a small ball (e.g., baseball) will be caught with one hand. However, as one grows hand size from childhood to adulthood, a ball previously caught with two hands (e.g., basketball) could now be caught with one hand. Therefore, the relationship between the ball size and hand size is relative and dynamic. The changing relationship changes the affordance information, consequently, different perceptions and actions were seen. Zhu and colleagues (2009, 2010, 2011) systematically studied the perceptual ability of selecting the optimal object for long-distance throwing. By manipulating the size and weight of throwing objects, they found that skilled throwers could always identify the best objects for throwing even if they varied in size and weight, which impacted the throwing biomechanics for each individual thrower. Interestingly, when skilled throwers were asked to compare these identified objects to judge how heavy they were, these objects were perceived to be equally heavy, suggesting that the affordance information for throwing is relative and remains unchanged for each thrower. Let's go back to our previous example of soccer goalkeeping skill, a successful action produced by a goalie to stop a goal will now require attention to the following cues that will enable perception of affordance information:

- The opening and height of the goal
- The arm and leg length of the goalie
- The posture of the goalie

- The posture of the kicker
- The ball velocity, trajectory, spin, and direction
- The style of kicking
- The cognitive and motor capabilities of the goalie (e.g., visual search pattern, ability to jump to different directions)

Compared to the previous list of perceptual cues based on the IP theory, the EA-based list appears to be more comprehensive and inclusive, inviting the goalie to draw relationships among relevant cues from both internal and external factors.

How to quantify movement preparation?

Knowing that perception must be involved in movement preparation (either determines or interacts with action), one might wonder how this process can be measured and quantified. Motor behaviorists have been using chronological measures to quantify movement preparation based on the assumption that it must take time for a "meaning" to be attached to the sensory information. Specifically, the movement preparation can be measured and quantified by the reaction time (RT), which is defined as a brief time lag between the presentation of a stimulus and the initiation of a response. Correspondingly, the movement time (MT) can be defined as the duration for a planned action to be completed, which marks the start and end of a response (Henry, 1961). Then, the sum of RT and MT constitutes total response time (TRT), which is typically used to quantify the speed of movement. For instance, a 100 m sprinter is timed from the moment the starting signal (e.g., gunshot) is given to the last step s/he touches or crosses the finish line, which should include an RT reflecting how long it took the sprinter to react to the starting signal by initiating the launch from the block, and an MT reflecting how long it took the sprinter to complete the running course. Accordingly, the training of 100 m sprint should involve both perceptual training focused on reducing the RT and physical training focused on reducing MT as reflected in Figure 5.1. Since the demands of RT and MT vary among different sport skills, the proportions of perceptual and physical training also vary depending on the sport skill to be learned.

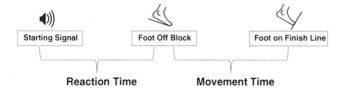

Figure 5.1 The Reaction Time (RT) and Movement Time (MT) in the example of 100m sprint.

For those practitioners who are helping students or athletes better prepare for the movement, a reduced RT would indicate that they have developed sufficient knowledge and a good perception about the motor skill and are ready to perform the skill. Otherwise, an increased RT would suggest that students or athletes have encountered some perceptual problems that prevented them from performing the skill efficiently. Then, what could have caused the perceptual problems to slow down the reaction? A list of five possible reasons are discussed next.

Number of response choices

The first possible reason is the number of response choices. If each stimulus corresponds to a response, then responding to only one stimulus will be much easier and faster than responding to one of many stimuli. This has been proven true by Hick (1952) who experimentally measured choice RT by manipulating the number of stimulus-response alternatives (choice or amount of uncertainty). The choice RT was found to be logarithmically related to the number of response choices in that there was a fixed amount of RT increment every time the number of response choices was doubled. The response uncertainty simply increased with the increasing number of response choices. In other words, the decision becomes harder when we are faced with many choices. As in the case of driving a car from a rural area into a metropolitan area, the driver's reaction to the yellow flash of traffic lights would be slower due to having to pay extra attention to the surrounding vehicles and pedestrians. Therefore, in teaching a motor skill with multiple skill cues, presenting all skill cues to students at once and asking students to use them may cause perceptual problems, resulting in an increased RT or delayed response.

Anticipation

The second possible reason is anticipation. In responding to a sequence of stimuli unfolding over time, if the performer has advance knowledge of what stimulus will be presented and when it will show itself, a better preparation of movements and a reduced RT are expected. Such an anticipation skill is often seen in elite athletes. Research has shown that elite tennis players can predict the opponent's stroke by watching the opponent's motion before ball contact so that their returns are faster and more accurate (Triolet et al., 2013). Therefore, the perceptual training focused on reducing RT should include developing the ability of anticipation. The performer should be not only informed of what and where the stimulus will appear (spatial anticipation), but also aware of when the expected stimulus will arrive (temporal anticipation).

Foreperiod consistency

The third possible reason is the foreperiod consistency. In developing the temporal anticipation, the consistency of foreperiod matters. The foreperiod is defined as the interval between the presentation of a warning signal and the stimulus (Niemi & Näätänen, 1981). If a highly expected stimulus never shows at the expected time, the anticipation will fail, and a delayed response will be seen. Therefore, tennis players often change the ball tossing height, thus, the duration of serve, to prevent their serves from being anticipated by their opponents.

Psychological refractory period

The fourth possible reason is the psychological refractory period. When two stimuli are presented in short succession, the response to the firstly presented stimulus will not be affected, while the response to the secondly presented stimulus will be significantly delayed. Such a phenomenon was reported by Davis (1956) and then referred to as psychological refractory period (PRP). PRP has a focus on the temporal structure of presenting sequential stimuli, suggesting that a bottleneck of information processing will be encountered if one stimulus is presented shortly after the other and both are demanding a quick response, in which the processing of future stimulus must wait until the completion of processing the current stimulus. The mechanism of PRP helped explain why the fake motions seen in sports often work. As seen in Figure 5.2 below, a typical fake motion will be presented right before the actual motion to elicit a response from the opponent, so that the response to the actual motion will be significantly delayed than that if without having the fake motion earlier. Therefore, to help students or athletes better prepare for the movements, teachers or coaches must help them discern the task-relevant stimulus from those distracting stimuli that may be intentionally presented to elicit earlier reactions.

Stimulus-response compatibility

The stimulus-response compatibility refers to the extent to which a stimulus and its required response are "naturally" related (Umiltá & Nicoletti, 1990).

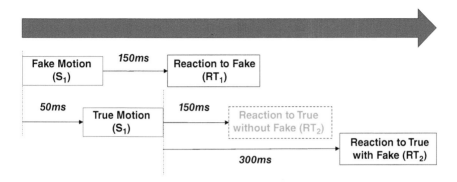

Figure 5.2 Task relevant Stimulus.

Here, the naturalness corresponds to a small RT because the minimum processing is needed. A stimulus can be naturally related to a response if they are spatially compatible. For instance, an instructor teaching an aerobics class often uses a large wall mirror to teach the sequential movements because the produced movements of the instructor and students are seen spatially compatible in the mirror, therefore, there is less delay for students to follow the instructor's movements. Such a S-R compatibility could be developed through practice as well. We all learned how to interpret the three colors of a traffic light (RED for "stop", YELLOW for "proceed with caution", and GREEN for "go") so that our response to the traffic light won't be delayed. However, if the law enforced the change of meaning for each colored light (e.g., RED for "go" and GREEN for "stop"), the delayed or mistaken responses will lead to a traffic disaster. Therefore, to help students better prepare for the movements, the practitioner must help students to relate a relevant stimulus to the specific response, establishing the S-R compatibility.

Attention and movement preparation

Perceptual problems emerged in movement preparation are often associated with the performer's limited knowledge about the relevant cues which also makes them susceptible to distraction from the irrelevant cues. In cognitive psychology, attention is defined as a process of selecting relevant cues while ignoring irrelevant cues for processing (Posner, 1988), and the influence of attention on motor performance has been well documented (Wulf, 2007). A motor skill with multiple relevant cues will require multiple attentional resources to sustain the performance; however, the overall attentional resources available for an individual are thought to have a fixed capacity (Bundesen, 1990). Therefore, degraded performance is expected if the fixed attentional capacity is run out and fails to support the selection of all relevant cues for processing. Although the individual attentional capacity is fixed, the attentional demands, that is, the attentional resources required for sustaining the performance, may vary depending on the environment, task, and the performer. The attentional demands will be high if the skill is performed in an open environment, complex involving many skill cues, or completely novel to the performer. Therefore, teaching a complex motor skill to novices should consider limiting the environmental changes and reducing the number of skill cues given for focus, so that the attentional demands can be reduced to a manageable level for the performer. To determine the attentional demands encountered by an individual, the dual-task paradigm is often used, which involves using a secondary task to probe the primary task (Karatekin et al., 2004). For example, to assess the attentional demands encountered by a volleyball setter during the setting task, we can set the primary task as setting the ball to a target area predetermined by the teacher or coach, and the secondary task as verbally responding to an auditory tone played in different phases of setting: (a) when the ball was tossed; (b) before the tossed ball reached its peak; (c) after the tossed ball reached its peak; or (d) before contacting the ball with hands. If the performance of the primary task, that is, the setting accuracy, dropped due to the influence of the secondary task in a probing phase, the attentional demand in that phase must be high for that setter. Otherwise, a well-maintained performance of the primary task in the presence of the secondary task would suggest a low attentional demand for that setter. To be noted, the dual-task paradigm is not only used to assess the attentional demands encountered by an individual, but also to train an individual to increase his/her fixed attentional capacity.

Regarding how attention would impact motor performance, a two-dimensional model of attention has been proposed to account for how attention can be used dynamically to support motor performance. According to Nideffer (1976), attention can be paid externally/internally and broadly/narrowly at the same time. Consequently, there are four types of attention that would impact both preparation and execution of movements as reflected in Table 5.1. The external-broad attention directs the performer to search the external environment for any cue that might be relevant to the motor task, which is required for assessing external environment; the external-narrow attention directs the performer to search the external environment for the specific cues relevant to the motor task, which is required for performing motor response; the internal-narrow attention directs the performer to search within mind and body for the specific cues relevant to the motor task, which is required for rehearsing an upcoming performance; and the internal-broad attention directs the performer to search within mind and body for any cue that might be relevant to the motor task, which is required for analyzing and planning strategy.

In sport psychology, attention is related to arousal which can be defined as a psychophysiological activation of the organism that varies from deep sleep to intense excitement (Gould & Krane, 1992). It was hypothesized that the relationship between motor performance and the level of arousal follows an inverted-U shape, in which a moderate level of arousal corresponds to the

Table 5.1 Nideffer's Two-dimensional Model of Attention

	External	
	Assessing offense and defense	Focusing on the person you are defending
Broad		**Narrow**
	Assessing fatigue, organizing complex serial response	Focusing on one aspect of response: fingertips, legs
	Internal	

Table 5.2 Strategies for increasing and decreasing arousal levels

Increase arousal level	Decrease arousal level
Increase rhythm/rate of breathing	Encourage slow and controlled breathing
Listen to upbeat music	Progressive muscle relaxation
Increase physical activity	Replace negative thoughts with positive ones
	Visualize a positive outcome
	Focus on performance rather than outcome

peak performance. If the arousal level is too low, the attention is too broad so that both relevant and irrelevant cues are attended, however, if the arousal level is too high, the attention becomes too narrow so that even the relevant cues could be neglected. Therefore, one needs to adjust the arousal level to find the optimum at which the most relevant cues can be attended to and processed for preparation of movements.

Strategies to increase and decrease arousal levels

Some strategies for increasing and decreasing arousal levels have been suggested by researchers and practitioners (Martens, 2012; Weinberg & Gould, 2015). We have them tabulated below in Table 5.2. Teachers or coaches must realize that the effectiveness of those strategies may vary among individuals. Therefore, when implementing those strategies, their mindsets need to be flexible, thus selecting appropriate strategies based on the characteristics of individual students or athletes.

Summary

In this chapter, we introduced perception and attention as the two important cognitive processes involved in movement preparation. We contrasted the definitions of perception in theoretical frameworks of information processing and ecological approach. Reaction time was identified as the behavioral measure of movement preparation, and factors that will influence reaction time were discussed. Finally, the role of attention in preparation for successful movements was discussed.

Questions for reflection

- What is the difference in defining perception between information processing theory and ecological approach?
- What is affordance information? Can you provide an example of how people can perceive the affordance information?
- What are the factors that will influence movement preparation?
- How to determine the attentional demand encountered by an individual?
- What are practical strategies to increase and decrease arousal levels?

References

Bundesen, C. (1990). A theory of visual attention. *Psychological Review*, *97*(4), 523.

Davis, R. (1956). The limits of the "psychological refractory period". *Quarterly Journal of Experimental Psychology*, *8*(1), 24–38.

Downing, L. (2004). George Berkeley, *The Stanford Encyclopedia of Philosophy* (Fall 2021 Edition), Edward N. Zalta (ed.).

Gibson, J. J. (1977). The theory of affordances. *Hilldale, USA*, *1*(2), 67–82.

Gould, D., & Krane, V. (1992). The arousal–athletic performance relationship: Current status and future directions. In T. S. Horn (Ed.), *Advances in sport psychology* (pp. 119–142). Champaign, IL, USA: Human Kinetics Publishers.

Henry, F. M. (1961). Reaction time – Movement time correlations. *Perceptual and Motor Skills*, *12*(1), 63–66.

Hick, W. E. (1952). On the rate of gain of information. *Quarterly Journal of Experimental Psychology*, *4*, 11–26.

Karatekin, C., Couperus, J. W., & Marcus, D. J. (2004). Attention allocation in the dual-task paradigm as measured through behavioral and psychophysiological responses. *Psychophysiology*, *41*(2), 175–185.

Martens, R. (2012). *Successful coaching*. Champaign, IL, USA: Human Kinetics.

Nideffer, R. M. (1976). Test of attentional and interpersonal style. *Journal of Personality and Social Psychology*, *34*(3), 394.

Niemi, P., & Näätänen, R. (1981). Foreperiod and simple reaction time. *Psychological Bulletin*, *89*(1), 133–162.

Posner, M. I. (1988).Structures and function of selective attention. In T. Boll & B. K. Bryant (Eds.), *Clinical neuropsychology and brain function: Research, measurement, and practice* (pp. 173–202). American Psychological Association. https://doi.org/10.1037/10063-005

Simon, H. A. (1978). Information-processing theory of human problem solving. *Handbook of learning and cognitive processes*, *5*, 271–295.

Triolet, C., Benguigui, N., Le Runigo, C., & Williams, A. M. (2013). Quantifying the nature of anticipation in professional tennis. *Journal of Sports Sciences*, *31*(8), 820–830.

Umiltá, C., &Nicoletti, R. (1990). *Spatial stimulus-response compatibility*. In R. W. Proctor & T. G. Reeve (Eds.), *Stimulus-response compatibility: An integrated perspective* (pp. 89–116). North-Holland: Elsevier.

Vereijken, B., Whiting, H. T. A., & Beek, W. J. (1992). A dynamical systems approach to skill acquisition. *The Quarterly Journal of Experimental Psychology Section A*, *45*(2), 323–344.

Weinberg, S. R., & Gould, D. (2015). *Foundation of sport and exercise psychology* (6th ed.). Champaign, IL, USA: Human Kinetics.

Wulf, G. (2007). *Attention and motor skill learning*. Champaign, IL, USA: Human Kinetics.

Zhu, Q., & Bingham, G. P. (2010). Learning to perceive the affordance for long-distance throwing: Smart mechanism or function learning? *Journal of Experimental Psychology: Human Perception and Performance*, *36*(4), 862.

Zhu, Q., Dapena, J., & Bingham, G. P. (2009). Learning to throw to maximum distances: Do changes in release angle and speed reflect affordances for throwing? *Human Movement Science*, *28*(6), 708–725.

Zhu, Q., & Bingham, G. P. (2011). Human readiness to throw: The size–weight illusion is not an illusion when picking the best objects to throw. *Evolution and Human Behavior*, *32*(4), 288–293.

6 Theoretical approaches
Mechanisms underlying skilled movements

Outcomes

- Understand movement pattern and control variables required to sustain a movement pattern.
- Understand and differentiate the top-down and bottom-up control mechanisms.

A skilled movement must be well-controlled, then what can be controlled to make movements qualitatively different? Two motor control mechanisms have been proposed to account for the neural processes underlying skilled movements: the top-down and bottom-up control mechanisms (Tani, 2003). Although they approached the control mechanism differently, both have guided motor control research and teaching of motor skills.

Behavioral observation of motor control

It is often a trivial task for someone to tell one that movement is performed qualitatively differently than the other, and a consensus on the quality of movements can be easily reached among people too. Movement pattern is defined as the invariant way to organize movement components in time and space, which can be easily picked up by the eyes of the observer. However, multiple movement patterns exist because there are multiple ways of organizing movement components in time and space to achieve the goal. For instance, to pick up a pen on a table, one can reach toward the pen in a linear path and grasp it with the thumb and index finger or reach toward the pen in a cursive path and grasp it with any fingers. Both will work although we know that the former is normal and efficient, and the latter is awkward and redundant. Therefore, the process of becoming skilled is also the process of finding a movement pattern to achieve a specific goal with minimum effort and time. A skilled movement is also a coordinated movement. Coordination is a term used to describe the process of bringing different movement components into a proper spatiotemporal order to ensure efficiency. A motor skill is learned if the coordination required for the skill is developed.

Although a skilled movement is characterized by an invariant coordination pattern, each movement component involved in a skill has a range to vary

DOI: 10.4324/9781003331964-8

their values if they can be quantified, and these variable components are called control variables or parameters (Latash, 2010). For example, one can walk fast or slow without changing the coordination pattern of walking. In this case, the respective working durations of the muscles and joints involved in producing walking movements are just shortened without the relationship among them being changed in timing the entire movements. Therefore, the absolute time or force utilized for the relevant muscles to shorten/lengthen or the relevant joints to flex/extend/rotate constitutes control variables that can be changed within a range to sustain a pattern of movement.

The knowledge of movement pattern and control variables provides a behavioral tool for practitioners to observe how movement patterns can be qualitatively changed by changing the control variables, which will allow for designing and implementing behavioral intervention for skill acquisition. However, what has happened and what has caused that to happen before overt motor behavior can be observed? The knowledge of neural processes involved in producing movements is relevant. The internal models of motor control (Kawato & Wolpert, 2007) have suggested that two neural pathways (afferent and efferent) are responsible for voluntary control of movements, which leads to the two possible motor control mechanisms that will be introduced below.

Control mechanisms underlying skilled movements

Two mechanisms are available to account for the motor control of skilled movements. Although contradictory to one another, they are complementary to help with understanding the flexibility of motor control in dealing with the changing constraints of task and environment.

As illustrated in Figure 6.1, the human nervous system consists of the central nervous system (CNS, the brain and spinal cord) and peripheral nervous system (PNS, the nerves that carry impulses to and from the central nervous system) (Ordovas-Montanes et al., 2015). The two nervous systems are connected through Afferent and Efferent pathways. The former is transmitting sensory information from sensory organs to the central nervous system, while the latter is carrying motor information away from the central nervous system to the muscles and glands of the body. Considering that movement production is the result of working CNS and PNS, the control of movement could involve just the efferent pathway (so-called top-down control), or both afferent and efferent pathways (so-called bottom-up control) (McMains & Kastner, 2011).

Top-down control mechanism

The top-down control mechanism assumes that the CNS can prescribe motor commands and order the muscle and body to move merely via the efferent pathway. Evidence from both animal and human studies supported the existence

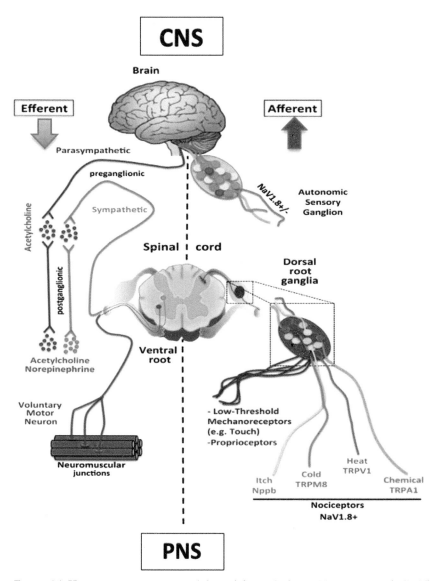

Figure 6.1 Human nervous system. Adapted from Ordovas-Montanes et al. (2015). The regulation of immunological processes by peripheral neurons in homeostasis and disease. *Trends in Immunology, 36*(10), 578–604.

Source: Copyright permission obtained.

of top-down control mechanisms. Taub and his colleagues (1966, 1975) reported that monkeys with deafferented (a surgical procedure to free a motor nerve from sensory components by severing the dorsal root central to the dorsal ganglion) forelimbs were still able to grasp and point accurately at visual targets with and without vision of their limbs. In performing voluntary rapid arm movement, the tri-phasic EMG activation pattern from the agonist and antagonist muscles remained unchanged even when the movement was unexpectedly blocked (Wadman et al., 1979), suggesting that the CNS governs the muscles responsible for fast movements before sensory feedback can join and impact the movement. The empirical results from both animal and human studies led to the formation and proposition of motor program theory (Schmidt, 1985), according to which, an abstract representation exists in the CNS that can be called upon for planning and organizing specific movements. The use of a motor program for motor control can be seen when performing a movement multiple times in various conditions, where some aspects of the movement remain unchanged while other aspects of the movement could be varied. Those that remain unchanged are invariant features including the sequence of action events, relative time and relative force. Those that can be varied are variant parameters including the selection of action effectors, overall time, and overall force. For instance, in playing soccer, one can shoot with dominant or non-dominant leg, fast or slow, but the sequence of joint action among hip, knee, and ankle and the duration of each joint action in relation to the duration of all joint actions remains unchanged. Such an invariant spatiotemporal pattern of sequential actions is often referred to as a kinematic chain. Since action is centrally prescribed to effectors without use of sensory inputs, the motor control based on motor program is open loop in nature. An open-loop control system runs fast and efficient because it saves the time required for processing the sensory inputs, this is particularly useful when there is a time constraint for a movement (e.g., throwing or kicking a ball under the pressure of opponents).

Bottom-up control mechanism

The bottom-up control mechanism includes both afferent and efferent pathways, therefore, closing the loop between CNS and PNS. In such a closed-loop system, the afferent/sensory information is not only required for planning of movement, but also feeds the consequence of movement back to the system for continuous refinement of movement in real time or the subsequent trial until a pre-determined goal is achieved. A variety of sensory receptors are available in our body to supply sensory information for motor control. Exteroceptors, such as receptors located in our eyes and ears, provide information regarding the external environment relevant to the movement, while proprioceptors, such as receptors located in our muscles, tendons, and joints, provide information regarding the body position and status of body movement. Both types of sensory information will be integrated in the CNS before a motor command is formed and issued to the corresponding effector, such sensory integration and motor command issuing will continue until the goal of movement is achieved.

In fact, the bottom-up control mechanism attaches great importance to sensory integration so that the role of motor command issuing is minimal and could be ignored. Since the afferent information is instantaneously accessed via the sensory receptors and the movement production will be based on the updated afferent information, there is no need for use of a motor program, which could be outdated, for motor control. Therefore, the movement pattern can be instantaneously adjusted to meet the changing demands of the task. This control mechanism is consistent with the view of the dynamic interaction theory of motor control (Davids et al., 2003), according to which, a patterned movement is self-organized, as opposed to being programed, by virtual of perceiving the constraints imposed by actor, task, and environment. This theory is also supported by evidence from both animal and human studies. In a study of horse gait patterns and the associated energetics as a function of locomoting speed, Hoyt and Taylor (1981) reported that horse switched the gait patterns (walking, trotting, and galloping) to maintain minimal energy expenditure in response to the increasing speed of locomotion. Later, in an experiment where human subjects were asked to maintain an anti-phase pattern of rhythmic bimanual finger tapping while gradually increasing their speed of movement (Kelso, 1984), a spontaneous switch from the anti-phase pattern to the in-phase pattern was observed at a threshold speed, even though it was not intended. Both studies have suggested that a patterned movement emerges, rather than being planned, to deal with the changing demand of the task that was intrinsically perceived.

In the constraints-led approach to skill acquisition (Davids et al., 2008), constraints are defined as the factors that both limit and enable movement solutions, which are imposed by actor, task, and environment. The actor constraints refer to the biological and functional characteristics of the actor including the dimension, strength, and conditioning of the body, as well as the level of cognition the actor possesses. The task constraints refer to the motor task including the required equipment, rules, and goals. Environmental constraints refer to any environmental factor that may affect motor performance such as light, temperature, and gravity. Although each type of constraint may influence the movement, only an interaction among these three types of constraints will specify a movement pattern, which is supported by the afferent pathway carrying rich sensory information. For instance, basketball players often switch between two-hand throw and one-hand throw during play. If the player has a hand size allowing for a full grasp of the ball with one hand (interaction between actor constraint and task constraint), and the distance between the player's position and the basket is also short allowing for a layup (interaction between environmental constraint and actor constraint), the one-hand throw is more likely to be seen than two-hand throw, and vice versa. Hence, the movement solution is self-organized and presenting itself as the constraints unfold, rather than being pre-programed like the top-down control mechanism assumes.

As indicated earlier, the two motor control mechanisms introduced above shall be treated as complementary rather than contradictory because they both are supported by empirical evidence collected from animal and human studies, each representing a possibility for movement production. It may well be possible that both control mechanisms are involved in developing skilled movements, considering that the sensory feedback is required in early skill acquisition, while its role is diminished in later skill acquisition since the motor program-based control is more efficient in supporting the control of skilled movements that often come with a time constraint.

Summary

In this chapter, we first define movement pattern and control variables, which provides a behavioral tool for practitioners to observe the control of movements. Then, we introduce two motor control mechanisms that can account for the neural processes involved in producing and controlling movements. Although the two mechanisms are contrasting with respect to the role of afferent information in motor control, we conclude that these two control mechanisms could be complementary to help understand the flexibility of motor control in dealing with the changing constraints of task and environment.

Questions for reflection

- What is movement pattern and what are control variables that will be required to sustain a movement pattern?
- What are the two neural pathways involved in neuromotor control according to the internal model?
- What is the Top-down control mechanism? What is the Bottom-up control mechanism? And how to differentiate them?

References

Davids, K., Button, C., & Bennett, S. (2008). *Dynamics of skill acquisition: A constraints-led approach*. Champaign, IL, USA: Human kinetics.

Davids, K., Glazier, P., Araújo, D., & Bartlett, R. (2003). Movement systems as dynamical systems. *Sports Medicine*, *33*(4), 245–260.

Hoyt, D. F., & Taylor, C. R. (1981). Gait and the energetics of locomotion in horses. *Nature*, *292*(5820), 239–240.

Kawato, M., & Wolpert, D. (2007, September). Internal models for motor control. In *Novartis foundation symposium 218: Sensory guidance of movement* (pp. 291–307). Chichester, UK: John Wiley & Sons, Ltd.

Kelso, J. A. (1984). Phase transitions and critical behavior in human bimanual coordination. *American Journal of Physiology-Regulatory, Integrative and Comparative Physiology*, *246*(6), R1000–R1004.

Latash, M. L. (2010). Motor synergies and the equilibrium-point hypothesis. *Motor Control*, *14*(3), 294–322.

McMains, S., & Kastner, S. (2011). Interactions of top-down and bottom-up mechanisms in human visual cortex. *Journal of Neurosciences*, *31*(2), 587–597.

Ordovas-Montanes, J., Rakoff-Nahoum, S., Huang, S., Riol-Blanco, L., Barreiro, O., & von Andrian, U. H. (2015). The regulation of immunological processes by peripheral neurons in homeostasis and disease. *Trends in Immunology*, *36*(10), 578–604.

Schmidt, R. A. (1985). The 1984 CH McCloy research lecture: The search for invariance in skilled movement behavior. *Research Quarterly for Exercise and Sport*, *56*(2), 188–200.

Tani, J. (2003). Learning to generate articulated behavior through the bottom-up and the top-down interaction processes. *Neural Networks*, *16*(1), 11–23.

Taub, E., Ellman, S. J., & Berman, A. J. (1966). Deafferentation in monkeys: Effect on conditioned grasp response. *Science*, *151*(3710), 593–594.

Taub, E., Goldberg, I. A., & Taub, P. (1975). Deafferentation in monkeys: Pointing at a target without visual feedback. *Experimental Neurology*, *46*(1), 178–186.

Wadman, W. J., Denier Van der Gon, J. J., Geuze, R. H., & Mol, C. R. (1979). Control of fast goal-directed arm movements. *Journal of Human Movement Studies*, *5*(1), 3–17.

7 Knowledge of learners

Outcomes

- Understand and contrast different models of stages of learning.
- Understand the relationship between Motor Learning and Motor Performance.
- Understand how to measure motor performance for the purpose of assessing motor learning.

In the ecological perspective of skill acquisition, the interaction among learner, task, and environment must happen before a motor skill can be learned. While task and environment are ever-changing factors that can be controlled and manipulated by teachers and coaches, learner is a factor that varies in the long term without the immediate changes that can be made by practitioners. Nevertheless, the learner's cognitive and motor abilities are evolving over time through education and experience, which is an enduring and irreversible process. Therefore, in designing practice for skill acquisition, the practitioners must be aware of the learner's status quo of learning and change the task and environmental factors accordingly to facilitate the learner's skill acquisition. In this chapter, we will focus on two questions: (1) how many stages of learning a learner must go through before fully mastering a motor skill? (2) how to assess motor learning?

Stages of learning

"Rome wasn't built in a day", same as with skill acquisition. It often takes multiple stages of learning to learn a complex motor skill. For instance, walking is so trivial for us as an adult, but it did take years for us to master this skill: One must first develop the ability to stand upright with two feet, the ability to alternate the stance and swing legs, and then the ability to coordinate the upper and lower limbs to keep balance while locomoting. Apparently, during each stage of learning how to walk, there are skill cues that the learner needs to attend and receive feedback on from teachers or coaches, based on which specific instructional activities can be designed and offered to facilitate learning. Therefore, identifying the stage of learning will help teachers or coaches to understand the needs (instructional or psychological) of learners

DOI: 10.4324/9781003331964-9

throughout the learning process, and then to determine the appropriate learning tasks and instructional activities.

In the literature of motor learning, two models of stages of learning are known to impact practical teaching and coaching of motor skills, which are: Fitts and Posner's 3-stage model (1967) and Gentile's 2-stage model (Schmidt et al., 2018).

Fitts and Posner's 3-stage model

This is a classic model proposed by Fitts and Posner (1967) for understanding of human performance and learning. There are three sequential stages one must go through before a superior performance can be demonstrated: cognitive stage, associative stage, and autonomous stage. During the cognitive stage, the learners develop a fundamental pattern of movement by figuring out the required action components. They keep thinking and asking questions and use a trial-and-error approach to solve movement problems. Their motor performance is marked with many errors and a high variability. They need teachers or coaches around to offer guidance, detect errors, and provide solutions to correct errors. During the associative stage, the learners are committed to refining the established fundamental pattern of movement by linking the required action components identified from the previous stage. Learners use comparative and associative analyses to differentiate and connect all required action components, so the movement organization and production become more successful. Their motor performance is improved with fewer errors and more consistency. Although their ability to detect and correct errors by themselves has improved, learners need teachers or coaches who can provide structured practice and constructive feedback to advance the skill. Finally, in the autonomous stage, the learners are no longer engaged in cognitive processing and the movement organization and execution become automatic without the need of attention or effort from the learners. While the motor performance is featured with minimum error and high consistency, the learners are confident and even capable of multitasking. Their ability to detect and correct errors continues to improve so that learners can even help others to detect and correct errors. However, the learners may become discouraged and unmotivated if they perceive their performance to stop advancing or advance slower than they expected. Therefore, learners need teachers or coaches around who can continue to provide support and motivate them to practice if motor expertise is demanded. For example, in learning one-hand dribbling in basketball, students or athletes at the cognitive stage will ask more questions than doing. Should they push down the ball when the ball is coming up or going down? Even if students or athletes were told that they should push down the ball when the ball is coming up at its peak, they would still have a hard time keeping the ball bouncing up and down continuously. As students or athletes progress to the associate stage, they will focus on performing the task, although they would ask the teachers or coaches if a certain strategy they developed through practice, such as matching the hand movement with ball movement or using palm instead of fingers to push down the ball, should be maintained or discarded. Finally, students or athletes at the autonomous stage will be able to perform the one-hand dribbling independently and reliably without need to consult with the teachers or coaches, however, they will need the teachers or coaches to introduce some new constraints to challenge their skill, such as, one-hand dribbling with walking or running.

Gentile's 2-stage model

Gentile (1972) proposed a working model for skill acquisition that has influenced the practical coaching and teaching of motor skills for decades. According to Gentile, there are only two stages for skill acquisition. The first stage is termed as getting the idea of the movement, during which the learners are committed to developing the basic movement pattern by discriminating between regulatory and non-regulatory conditions. The regulatory conditions refer to task constraints including the required action components, rules, equipment, and goals, while the non-regulatory conditions refer to environmental constraints including light conditions, room or outdoor temperature, and background noise. Cognitive processing is heavily involved in this stage as the learners are trying to identify what's relevant and irrelevant, as well as to figure out how relevant cues can be combined for successful movement production. To facilitate the understanding, the readers may consider Gentile's first stage of learning as a combination of cognitive and associative stages in Fitts and Posner's 3-stage model.

However, what makes Gentile's model unique is her second stage of learning, which is termed as fixation/diversification. In this stage, the learners are committed to refining a motor skill based on the basic movement pattern developed from the previous stage. However, skill refinement is achieved with two different types of practice depending on the nature of the skill being learned. "Fixation" refers to using constant practice for skill refinement if the skill being learned falls in the category of closed skills. In other words, if the environment in which the skill will be performed is relatively stable (e.g., 100-meter sprint), the skill refinement should involve a lot of repetitions of movement so that the invariant movement pattern can be developed. In contrast, "Diversification" refers to using variable practice for skill refinement if the skill being learned falls in the category of open skills. In other words, if the environment in which the skill will be performed is ever changing (e.g., playing basketball), the skill refinement should involve practicing the skill in variant conditions that best simulate the changing environment, so that the developed movement pattern can be adapted to different situations to deal with the changing environmental demands.

Since the stages of learning are directly associated with practice methods, Gentile's model has gained much popularity among practitioners. For instance, in learning how to serve a tennis ball, students or athletes must get an idea that the skill involves three movements: tossing the ball up, winding up the racquet, and striking the ball overhead. The key to success is that the served ball must fly over the net and land inside the service box on the opposite side of the court. Therefore, the control of striking angle and speed during the ball-racquet contact is the key skill component. Based on this idea, should the following practice be focused on Fixation or Diversification? Considering that tennis players often change the ball tossing height, speed of racquet swing, and striking point to make their serves unpredictable by the opponent (an open skill in nature), diversification should be recommended for the player in the next stage to refine the skill, which means the player should practice the serve by varying the tossing height, speed of swinging racquet, and the striking point.

Similarities and differences between two models

As mentioned earlier, the two models are similar because both agree that: (1) a task-specific cognitive processing must precede any motor production; (2) motor learning involves a shifting of focus from cognitive thinking to motor production. However, the two models differ largely in what happens after the completion of cognitive processing. While Fitts and Posner's 3-stage model considers that motor production based on the established cognitive representation of skill is merely automatic, Gentile's 2-stage model specifies the method for refining the motor production, which embraces the idea that functional movements are shaped by interactions among task, environment, and the actor.

In practical use of different models of stages of learning, we should be cautious of three things. First, although multiple learning stages are defined in different models, the transition between different learning stages cannot be clearly delineated. Often, one stage will blend into the next. For instance, elite athletes may still consult with the coach about some strategies that might help with enhancing their performances, indicating the continuous effort of associative learning in the autonomous stage. Second, a learner can be in different stages in learning different skills. One can be in the early stage of learning swimming, while at an advanced level in playing basketball. Finally, stages of learning are not dependent on age, but on the accumulated amount of practice. Although ages are typically correlated with the accumulated amount of practice, there are cases where one has accumulated a significant amount of practice in early age due to early specialization, or one has no accumulated amount of practice in late ages due to no prior exposure to certain skill before.

Assessing motor learning

Motor learning is defined as a process of acquiring a relatively permanent capability to perform certain movements (Schmidt et al., 2018). Therefore, the assessment of motor learning should focus on detecting the change of capability

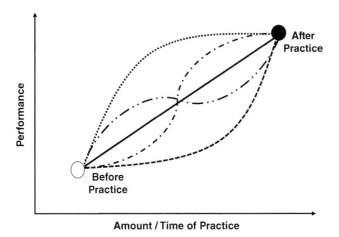

Figure 7.1 Performance curves as a function of practice. Pay attention that the same amount of practice yielded different ways of improving performance (both linear and non-linear) to achieve the same level of performance in the end!

to perform a movement, and make sure that the detected change is relatively permanent. As illustrated in Figure 7.1, the same amount of practice could yield different ways of improving performance (both linear and non-linear) to achieve the same level of skill proficiency due to individual differences in responding to the practice.

Yet, one's motor performance changes not only because of practice-induced motor learning, but also because it's subject to temporary factors such as motivation, fatigue, and arousal level of the nervous system. To assess motor learning, the change of motor performance due to the temporary factors needs to be removed, so that only the change due to practice remains. Typically, the learner's motor performance during practice needs to be measured multiple times and monitored to allow for the identification of positive change of performance.

In addition, a retention test should be followed, during which the motor performance can be reassessed to compare with the performance achieved at the end of the practice. This will not only allow for the effect of temporary factors on motor performance to dissipate, but also make sure the changed performance due to practice is relatively permanent. For example, during a practice session of basketball free throws, one student or athlete reported to a teacher or coach saying that he/she improved the throwing accuracy from 2 out 10 throws (20%) to 8 out of 10 throws (80%). Knowing that the reported performance enhancement might be related to some temporary factors such as the student's motivation and accidental use of correct throwing technique, the teacher or coach may ask the student or athlete to demonstrate the skill in the next practice session the next day, and the solid motor learning occurred during original practice can be only confirmed if the student's or athlete's throwing accuracy could be maintained to be close to 80%.

There are many ways to measure motor performance, which will allow for inference of motor learning. Traditionally, motor performance is measured by movement outcomes (e.g., speed, accuracy, score) due to the convenience and easy access to the measuring device. However, with the advancement of technology, motor performance can be quantified and assessed not only based on the product but also on the process of movement. For instance, practice could result in the change of movement organization from freezing degrees of freedom to freeing degrees of freedom, which can be seen with the increased range of motion at the relevant joints. Therefore, videotaping the movement and sequentially tracking the lines connecting all relevant joints will allow for visual examination of the development of range of motion (see Figure 7.2).

Similarly, practice could result in more fluid muscle activities during movement, therefore, using electromyography sensors to measure and monitor muscle activities on the involved muscles and detect the spatial-temporal change of signals as a function of practice would allow for assessment of the development of neuromuscular control of motor skill. In an aiming task that required a rapid elbow extension, Gabriel (2002) examined the variability of kinematic and EMG data as a function of practice. As seen in Figure 7.3, a high variability of kinematic data corresponded to a high variability of EMG data collected on Biceps and Triceps in early practice trials, however, the variability of both kinematic and EMG data reduced in late practice trials,

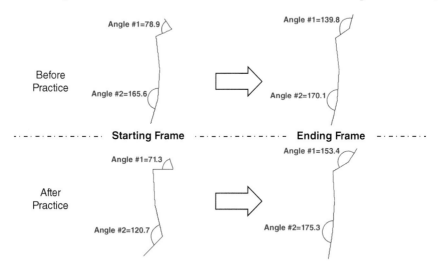

Figure 7.2 Illustration of the change of range of motion at elbow and knee for basketball throw through practice. Motion was captured in the sagittal plane with major joints (wrist, elbow, shoulder, hip, knee, and ankle) highlighted for visual tracking of joint (elbow and knee) angle changes from the start to the end of the movement both before and after the practice.

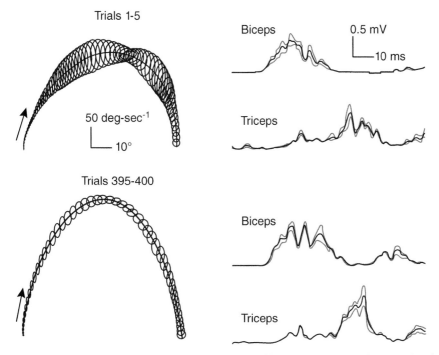

Figure 7.3 The corresponding reduction of variability in kinematic and EMG data in practicing a targeted maximal elbow flexion task.

Source: Copyright permission obtained.

suggesting that practice resulted in greater central nervous system control over the spatial-temporal pattern of both muscle (biceps and triceps) activation and movement trajectory.

The recent development of biosensor technology is enabling more sophisticated bio-signals (e.g., ECG, EMG, EEG) related to motor control to be measured and monitored for detection of biobehavioral changes in response to the practice aimed for skill acquisition. By combining the traditional movement outcome measures with the movement process measures, the practice-induced motor learning can be detected earlier and thoroughly. In a recent study (Wang et al., 2023), air pistol athletes' psychophysiological state during the aiming and firing periods were measured by EEG and ECG, and then correlated with shot performance, where "≥10.0 ring" was considered successful performance. It was found that the ability to maintain the brain–cardiac system at a benign dual activation level during the aiming and firing period would lead to successful shot performance, and the athletes' EEG and ECG have the trend to be synchronized approaching the firing time in successful performance as well. Accordingly, monitoring and detecting the psychophysiological state change of pistol athletes in response to practice can help with early detection of motor learning and predicting their successful performance.

Alternatively, motor learning can be accessed using cognitive and psychological measures. Since motor learning will lead to improved task-specific knowledge, memory, self-confidence, attention, and the ability to detect and correct errors, one can use standard knowledge tests and psychological questionnaires or scales to assess learners on these constructs at different stages of learning to estimate the progression of motor learning. To be noted, the ability to pay attention can also be objectively measured using eye-tracking technology.

Numerous studies on visual search and motor performance (Vickers, 2009) have shown that skilled performers can direct attention to relevant areas, pay a wide attention to the external environment, and switch attention between different tasks; while beginners often have difficulty finding the relevant cues, pay a narrowed attention to their body movement, and have inflexibility to switch attention. Therefore, motor learning can be inferred from the qualitative change of visual search patterns detected by tracking the learners' eye movements.

Summary

In this chapter, we first introduce two models of stages of learning and their applications for practitioners to assess the learner's skill level and their instructional needs. Then, we focus on defining and assessing motor learning, in which different measures of motor performance are introduced and how changes of those performance measures can inform motor learning is discussed.

Questions for reflection

- What are the three stages of learning specified in Fitts and Posner's model? What does the learner's motor behavior look like and what are their instructional needs at each stage?
- What are the two stages of learning specified in Gentile's model? How is Gentile's model similar and different from Fitts and Posner's model?
- What is the relationship between Motor Learning and Motor Performance?
- Can you raise two examples for motor performance being measured by process instead of by product?

References

Fitts, P. M., & Posner, M. I. (1967). *Human performance*. Brooks/Cole.

Gabriel, D. A. (2002). Changes in kinematic and EMG variability while practicing a maximal performance task. *Journal of Electromyography and Kinesiology, 12*(5), 407–412.

Gentile, A. M. (1972). A working model of skill acquisition with application to teaching. *Quest, 17*(1), 3–23.

Schmidt, R. A., Lee, T. D., Winstein, C., Wulf, G., & Zelaznik, H. N. (2018). *Motor control and learning: A behavioral emphasis.* Human kinetics.

Vickers, J. N. (2009). Advances in coupling perception and action: The quiet eye as a bidirectional link between gaze, attention, and action. *Progress in Brain Research, 174,* 279–288. Elsevier.

Wang, K., Li, Y., Liu, H., Zhang, T., & Luo, J. (2023). Relationship between Pistol Players' Psychophysiological State and Shot Performance: Activation Effect of EEG and HRV. *Scandinavian Journal of Medicine & Science in Sports, 33,* 84–98. 10.1111/sms.14253

8 Design task progressions

Outcomes

- Understand the definitions of task progressions, task, and task development.
- Understand and differentiate the concepts of informing, refining, extending, and applying task and understand how task develops in teaching physical education.
- Recognize the factors that affect task complexity.
- Be able to design teaching progressions by modifying the task complexity.

Definition of task

What is a task? In motor learning, a task is defined as a learning activity with a specific goal, and the procedures needed to achieve that goal (Magill & Anderson, 2021). For example, a motor learning task is when students or athletes are asked to kick a ball over a barrier and onto a targeted area for points. In this book, a task is defined as a unit of analysis. It can mean anything from knowledge, concept, and culture to sports skills being analyzed. A task can be either micro or macro in character. Using basketball as an example, possible micro tasks include the identification of the critical components in a layup skill, detection of skill errors, or designing an intervention to correct the errors. Possible macro tasks can be learning basketball history, culture, rules and etiquette, equipment, techniques, or offensive and defensive tactics.

Definition of task progressions

An effective teacher or coach must be able to design task progressions for all the tasks and subtasks in a sport. Task progressions are defined as a series of tasks sequenced in a progressive manner that moves students or athletes from the less complex and sophisticated to more difficult and complicated tasks by decreasing or increasing complexity. For example, when teaching or coaching a basketball chest-passing technique, a teacher or coach can start with an initial task for students or athletes to practice after instruction and demonstration, where

DOI: 10.4324/9781003331964-10

students or athletes in partner practice chest pass stationarily five feet apart. During practice, a teacher or coach can provide verbal feedback to improve technical proficiency of the chest pass or design a task for students or athletes to correct their technical errors. After students or athletes can successfully execute chest passes, a teacher or coach can move students or athletes to a more challenging task by extending the distance, where they in partner pass the ball while eight feet apart.

Conceptual framework for developing task progressions

The ability to develop task progressions is a critical skill for teachers or coaches to have since it is essential for them to implement instructions to achieve a specific instructional outcome (Rink, 1979, 2014; Ward, 2013). The development of task progressions is a process, where teachers or coaches select and sequence developmentally appropriate instructional tasks to meet the needs of learners for successful learning. The conceptualization of task development by Rink (1979) can be used as a framework to develop task progressions.

Rink (1979, 2014) conceptualized instructional task progressions as four different types of tasks: informing task, refining task, extension task, and application task. The informing task is an initial task in a sequence to teach a specific outcome. For example, in a football overhand throwing lesson or practice session, the first task that students or athletes practice is to throw the football with a partner while five feet apart. This task will be an informing task since it is the initial task in a sequence to teach students or athletes how to perform overhand throwing.

A task can be refined by focusing on the quality of the performance. The refining task is developed based on their observations of students' or athletes' performance and focuses on improving the technical proficiency of overhand throwing. The conditions of practice remain the same relative to the previous task. The focus of students' or athletes' attention will change as different technical elements are emphasized. For example, using the initial task of football overhand throwing, when students or athletes cannot keep the throwing elbow in an "L" shape, teachers or coaches can ask them to bring back the throwing arm and hold the elbow in an "L" shape position for multiple times to develop muscle memory. After the completion of this refining task, students or athletes can go back to practice the initial informing task in a complete full motion.

Teachers or coaches can extend a task by increasing or decreasing the complexity or difficulty levels relative to a previous task. Using the football initial informing task as an example, it can be extended by asking students or athletes to increase their distance from five feet to eight feet. This change in distance will present a challenge to students or athletes in terms of power or momentum generation and throwing accuracy. This initial informing task can also be extended by passing to a slow-moving partner. This extension task is more difficult as one must execute throwing relative to the moving speed of his or her practice partner.

An application task is a task which focuses on applying skills in more authentic ways. It provides an opportunity for students or athletes to apply the performance in a particular context or game. Using football overhand throwing as an example, an application task will be to have students play a 4-versus-4 modified game.

Factors affecting task complexity

The complexity of a task can be affected by numerous factors. Those factors include space and boundaries of the play area, equipment, number of players, timing, game rules, game conditions, tactics and problems, attacker/defender ratio, nature of the goal, and nature of the skills (closed versus open). For example, in soccer, dribbling with a defender in a small space is more difficult than dribbling with a defender in a larger space. In football, throwing a ball for a long distance will be more difficult than a short distance since a longer distance requires more strength and accuracy. In volleyball, a bigger and lighter ball is easier for kids than a regular ball. A bigger and lighter ball gives kids better control since their hands are small and arm muscles are not strong. In a 3v2 modified game, having one more offensive player will increase the difficulty for the two defensive players to defend the space and make it easier for the offensive players to attack the space and goal.

A sport skill can be classified as either an open skill or a closed skill. A closed skill is a skill performed in a fixed environment, where the performance conditions remain constant. An open skill is a skill performed in an ever-changing environment, where the performance conditions are variable (Magill & Anderson, 2021). For a closed skill, students or athletes will mainly focus on the technical demands that are performed invariably. However, for an open skill, students or athletes must adjust in relation to the changes in the relationship among environment, tasks, and individual. For example, in basketball, a jump shot without a defender in practice is easier to execute than a jump shot with a defender since students or athletes will have to adjust in relation to the movements of the defender. An open skill is more difficult to perform than a closed skill. By practicing a closed skill and then moving on to an open skill, teachers or coaches increase the difficulty of the practice.

How to develop task progressions

As stated earlier, task progressions are designed from less complex and difficult to more complex and difficult tasks by changing the factors that affect task complexity. Those progressions consist of a series of intertwined informing, refinement, extension, and application tasks that are arranged in a progressive manner to meet the needs of learners for better learning. In a typical coaching session or physical education lesson, task progressions start with an informing task, which is typically an easy, foundational learning task. During the practice of the informing task, teachers or coaches will use refinement tasks to improve students' or athletes' technical and/or tactical aspects of performance based on their observations. Upon the successful mastery of the informing task, teachers or coaches will use extension tasks to progress students' or athletes' performance by increasing the complexity of learning. During the practice of extension tasks, teachers or coaches will use refinement tasks to improve students' or athletes' technical and/or tactical aspects of performance based on their observations. Lastly, an application task will be used for students or athletes to transfer their learning into more authentic game situations. During the practice of the application task, teachers or coaches will use refinement tasks to improve students' or athletes' technical and/or tactical aspects of performance based on their observations. On the continuum of task progressions, the more complex and difficult tasks are more game-like, situational, and relational. By changing or combining characteristics of tasks in a skill, numerous progressions can be developed for skill development. The task complexity can also be increased by combining two or more skills to develop a task. The development of task progressions is like making a snowball, always increasing in size through added layers of snow.

For example, space can be increased or decreased to make soccer dribbling easier or more difficult. By adding more players, it can increase the complexity of a task since more options are available and more cognitive processing and decision making are needed for successful play performance. Moving from a closed skill to an open skill also makes a task more difficult. For example, a teacher or coach can start with 2 (players) versus 0 (no defenders) on chest passing in a 15 × 20 × 20 rectangle. After passing the ball, the player will need to move diagonally to an open corner. This is a closed skill where the emphasis will be on the technical elements of executing chest passing. For an open skill, a teacher or coach will spend less time on technical elements and more time on extending tasks that cover the variety of situations where the skill will be applied in games. To increase the difficulty and complexity, the teacher or coach can have students or athletes play a 2 (players) versus 1 (one defender) half-court game where the defensive player plays warm defense (following the offensive player with no stealing are allowed) and offensive players will be required to apply passing skills with at least four passes being made before they can shoot for a goal.

Table 8.1 presents a soccer dribbling for close control progression. The first progression is dribbling for close control with a back-away defender from the baseline to the midline. Having a defender ensures that the task presents a game-like scenario, and that the offensive player keeps his eyes up rather than looking at the ball, which is a common mistake students or players make. In the second and third progressions, having a defender step into the dribbling direction forces the offensive player to use cuts (inside, progression 2, or outside, progression 3) to change direction, which increases the difficulty. By adding turns and multiple defenders while allowing no stealing, progression 4 becomes more difficult, with more

Table 8.1 Progressive practices for soccer dribbling for close control

1 Dribble for close control with a back-away defender from one baseline to the midline
2 Dribble for close control with a defender stepping into the dribbling direction to force the dribbler to change direction using inside cut from one baseline to the midline
3 Dribble for close control with a defender stepping into the dribbling direction to force the dribbler to change direction using outside cut from one baseline to the midline
4 Dribble for close control using cuts and turns in a circle with defenders (no stealing)
5 Dribble for close control using cuts and turns in a circle with defenders actively stealing the ball
6 Use right foot roll across the ball and use left foot in-step to cut and get past a stationary defender
7 Use right foot roll across the ball and left foot in-step to cut and get past a warm defender
8 Use right foot roll across the ball and left foot in-step to cut and get past an active defender
9 Receive a pass and then use right foot roll across the ball and left foot in-step to cut and get past a stationary defender
10 Receive a pass and then use right foot roll across the ball and left foot in-step to cut and get pasts a warm defender
11 Receive a pass and then use right foot roll across the ball and left foot in-step to cut and get past an active defender
12 Use right foot roll across the ball and use left foot in-step to cut and get past a stationary defender, and then shoot for a goal
13 Use right foot roll across the ball and use left foot in-step to cut and get past a warm defender, and then shoot for a goal
14 Use right foot roll across the ball and use left foot in-step to cut and get past an active defender, and then shoot for a goal
15 Receive a pass, use right foot roll across the ball and use left foot in-step to cut and get past a stationary defender, and then shoot for a goal
16 Receive a pass, use right foot roll across the ball and use left foot in-step to cut and get past a warm defender, and then shoot for a goal
17 Receive a pass, use right foot roll across the ball and use left foot in-step to cut and get past an active defender, and then shoot for a goal

game-like elements. In progression 5, defenders are allowed to steal the ball. For progressions 6–8, dribbling techniques become more difficult with various degrees of defense, which enables students or players to become more skillful.

By adding other soccer skills such as passing and shooting, the rest of the progressions become more complex as more skills are involved. The progressive practices can get "bigger and bigger" by changing game parameters related to dribbling and passing as other skills are added. These progressive practices can move students or players successfully from one level to the next. Students or players can also easily apply them in games as these practices should be designed based on the scenarios taken from real games. Using a similar approach, Table 8.2 presents an example of progressive practices for a basketball chest pass. Due to space considerations, only partial progressive practices are listed in Tables 8.1 and 8.2.

Table 8.2 Progressive practices for basketball chest pass

1 Make a stationary pass and move to an open space: In a square with three players on three corners, pass a ball to one of the other two players and move to the open corner
2 Move and pass from middle line to baseline: Two players pass the ball back and forth while moving from midline to baseline
3 Make a stationary pass and move to an open space with a cold defender: In a square with three players on three corners, pass a ball to one of the other two players and move to the open corner. The defender will position in front of the ball player with hands up (no stealing)
4 Make a stationary pass and move to an open space with a warm defender: In a square with three players on three corners, pass a ball to one of the other two players and move to the open corner. The defender will move to block passing lane with hands moving up and down (no stealing)
5 Make a stationary pass and move to an open space with an active defender: In a square with three players on three corners, pass a ball to one of the other two players and move to the open corner. The defender will actively defend and try to steal the ball.
6 Move and pass from midline to baseline with a cold defender: Two players pass the ball back and forth while moving from midline to baseline. The defender positions his or her body close to the ball player and move back in the middle with no stealing
7 Move and pass from midline to baseline with a warm defender: Two players pass the ball back and forth while moving from midline to baseline. The defender positions his or her body close to the ball player and apply pressure but with no stealing
8 Move and pass from midline to baseline with an active defender: Two players pass the ball back and forth while moving from midline to baseline. The defender will defend the ball player actively with stealing.
9 2 versus 0: The ball player passes the ball to the other player, cuts to basket, receives the pass from the other player, and then shoots the basket (layup or jump shot).
10 2 versus 1: The ball player passes the ball to the other player, cuts to basket, receives the pass from the other player, and then shoots the basket (layup or jump shot). The defense will assume a stationary position to defend the ball player with hands up.
11 2 versus 1: The ball player passes the ball to the other player, cuts to basket, receives the pass from the other player, and then shoots the basket (layup or jump shot). The defense will assume a position to defend the ball player with warm defense by moving feet and hands (no stealing).
12 2 versus 1: The ball player passes the ball to the other player, cuts to basket, receives the pass from the other player, and then shoots the basket (layup or jump shot). The defense will actively defend the ball player with stealing.

Summary

This chapter discusses the definitions of task and task progressions. Rink's Conceptualization of task development can be used as a framework for developing task progressions. Teachers or coaches can use this conceptual framework to design task progressions by changing the complexity of tasks, thus improving students' or athletes' skill performances.

Questions for reflection

- What is a task?
- What is task progression?
- What is Rink's conceptualization of task development?
- What factors affect task complexity?

References

Magill, R., & Anderson, D. (2021). *Motor learning and control: Concepts and applications* (12th ed.). New York, NY: McGraw Hill.

Rink, J. (1979). *Development of a system for the observation of content development in physical education*. Unpublished doctoral dissertation. The Ohio State University.

Rink, J. (2014). *Teaching physical education for learning* (7th ed.). Boston, MA: McGraw-Hill.

Ward, P. (2013). The role of content knowledge in conceptions of teaching effectiveness in physical education. *Research Quarterly for Exercise and Sport, 84*, 431–440. 10.1080/02701367.2013.844045

Section 3

Biomechanical principles and applications to skill analysis

This section covers biomechanical concepts and principles and their applications to skill analysis with five chapters. Chapter 9 describes basic biomechanical concepts. Chapter 10 focuses on biomechanical principles in linear kinematics and their applications to skill analysis. Chapter 11 focuses on biomechanical principles in angular kinematics and their applications to skill analysis. Chapter 12 focuses on biomechanical principles in linear kinetics and their applications to skill analysis. Chapter 13 focuses on biomechanical principles in angular kinetics and their applications to skill analysis.

DOI: 10.4324/9781003331964-11

9 Introduction and basic biomechanical concepts

Outcomes

- Understanding the definitions and broad applications of biomechanics.
- Defining linear and angular motion and kinematics and kinetics.
- Evaluating the differences between scalars and vectors and between two-dimensional and three-dimensional motion.

Biomechanics

Biomechanics is an essential component of the kinesiology and physical education curriculum and has its unique advantages in understanding movements, identifying deficits, and guiding improvements (Hamill et al., 2015). Biomechanics is defined as "the study of the structure and function of biological systems by means of the methods of mechanics" (Hatze, 1974). Mechanics is the application of physics to analyze the motion and causes of motion of a physical object. Biomechanics focuses on the mechanical perspectives of biological systems. Within the context of kinesiology and physical education, we are mostly interested in understanding human movements, including but not limited to whole-body, joint, and segment movements, as well as bone and muscle motion. Several relevant subdisciplines include sports biomechanics for sports performance enhancement, injury biomechanics for injury prevention and rehabilitation, and applied biomechanics for solving applied problems.

Many performance outcomes are directly measured in mechanical variables. Examples include throwing distances, jumping heights, and time to complete a marathon or swimming race. The relationships among mechanical variables are determined by physical laws and equations, so a deterministic model can be developed among technical and performance variables. For example, the throwing distance of a ball is determined by two components: flight distance in a vacuum and lost/gained distance due to air resistance (Figure 9.1) (Chow & Knudson, 2011). In addition, the flight distance is determined by the release height, angle, and speed of the ball. Furthermore, the release height is defined by joint angles and segment lengths, while the release speed is determined by joint angular velocities and segment lengths.

DOI: 10.4324/9781003331964-12

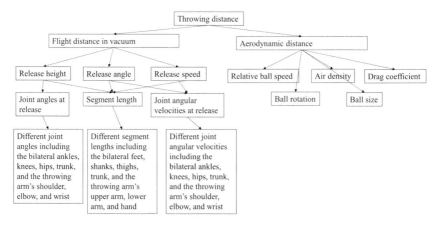

Figure 9.1 A biomechanical model of throwing distance.

By understanding the technical variables that can affect the performance outcome, we can target potential factors for improvements with the goal of enhancing performance. Other assessments, such as VO_2 max, body composition, and muscle strength, may have strong correlations with performance outcomes but may not explain 100% of the changes in performance.

While biomechanics may help identify movement errors, the improvement of performance typically involves more than biomechanical assessments. For beginners, some movement errors may be corrected by simple instruction and feedback. A novice volleyball player may be instructed to lower the body to pass the ball to gain better stability. A basketball player may be asked to land with more knee flexion for soft landings. However, the use of biomechanics for performance improvements in skilled athletes may be more challenging. For example, a coach may have identified a small release angle as a technical factor that limits a skilled thrower's throwing distance, but simply instructing the thrower to increase the release angle may not result in a longer throwing distance. It is possible the thrower can produce greater forces in the horizontal direction compared to the vertical direction, so the control strategy is self-optimized to have a small release angle for the longest distance. If the release angle is intentionally increased, the release speed may decrease and result in a decreased distance. A better strategy for this thrower might be increasing muscle force production in the vertical direction through strength training to increase the release angle without compromising release speeds. Another simple example could be distance running, the performance of which is affected by stride lengths (length of each stride) and stride frequencies (number of strides per minute). While it is straightforward that increasing stride frequencies with the same stride length will increase running speed, individuals may not be able to achieve this change throughout the race without improving VO_2 max and muscle endurance. In summary, biomechanics demonstrates its best value when used with other knowledge such as exercise physiology, motor control and learning, strength and conditioning, sports training, and coaching.

In summary, it is essential to understand the fundamental knowledge of biomechanics to analyze human movements. Compared to methods of "trial and error" and "best techniques", biomechanics can help evaluate individual differences and assess the advantages and limitations of certain techniques. Poor and problematic techniques can be explained to students in scientific languages. By identifying the contributing factors to the performance, we can also better break down the movements for intervention. Through appropriate data collection, the effects of technique modification and training on performance can be objectively quantified. For us to understand human movements, which can occur in both linear and angular forms, the first step is to describe how the object is moving. The next step is to understand the cause of the movement. As such, the next four sections categorize the analyses of human movements into the description and cause of linear and angular motion. In this chapter, we will introduce basic biomechanical terminologies.

Linear motion

All points on an object move the same distance without changing the object's orientation in linear motion (Hamill et al., 2015). Linear motion also occurs when the motion of a single point is analyzed since a single point does not have an orientation. For example, the seat of a moving wheelchair on an even surface is performing linear motion, as the orientation of the seat is not changing. The center of a ball is a single point, and its motion is considered linear motion.

Angular motion

The orientation of an object changes so that different points move through different distances in angular motion (Hamill et al., 2015). For example, the wheels of a moving wheelchair perform angular motion. While the center of a baseball is moving linearly, the other points of the baseball can rotate around the center in angular motion.

Kinematics

Kinematics is the description of the motion of an object without references to the cause of the motion (Hamill et al., 2015). For example, the athlete is running fast, and the ball has a high trajectory. The motion of the object is described without mentioning the cause of the fast speed or high trajectory.

Kinetics

Kinetics refers to the cause of the motion of an object (Hamill et al., 2015). For example, the athlete runs fast because he has strong leg muscles to generate a great amount of force. The ball has a high trajectory because the thrower has a strong arm to generate angular power. In these situations, the cause of the motion is described along with the description of the motion.

Scalar

Scalars are quantities with magnitudes but not directions (Hamill et al., 2015). Therefore, scalars can be fully described using numbers. Mass, volume, distance, and speed are scalars. For example, her mass is 50 kg, and the mass is fully described with the number without a direction associated with the mass. He ran 1,000 meters today. The 1,000-meter was described as a distance since there was no direction associated with it.

Vector

Vectors are quantities that describe both magnitudes and directions (Hamill et al., 2015). An arrow is commonly used to describe a vector. The length of the vector indicates the magnitude, and the way it is pointing gives the direction. Weight, displacements, and velocities are vectors. For example, her weight is 500 N, and the direction of the weight is pointing downward. He ran 1,000 meters to the north today. The 1,000-meter was described as a displacement since there was a direction. Figure 9.2 shows the magnitudes and directions of ground reaction forces in a forward jump.

Two-dimensional motion

Two-dimensional motion refers to the motion that mainly occurs in two directions in a single plane. For example, most running motion occurs in the anterior-posterior and vertical directions. Most jumping-jack motion occurs in the medial-lateral and vertical directions. The trunk motion in Hula Hoop activities mainly occurs in the anterior-posterior and medial-lateral directions. The long jump, standing vertical jump, and medicine ball throwing primarily involve two-dimensional motion. Two-dimensional motion is typically described using a two-dimensional Cartesian coordinate with the right and upward directions as positive x and y directions (Figure 9.3). The center of the coordinate is the origin, with both x and y being 0. The unit of the coordinate is determined by the variable to be measured.

Three-dimensional motion

Three-dimensional motion refers to the motion that occurs in three directions. For example, a running and cutting movement involved running in the anterior-posterior direction, turning the body in the medial-lateral direction, and lowering and raising the body in the vertical direction. Three-dimensional motion is typically described using a three-dimensional Cartesian coordinate with the right, forward, and upward directions as positive x, y, and z directions (Figure 9.3). The origin defines all x, y, and z to be 0.

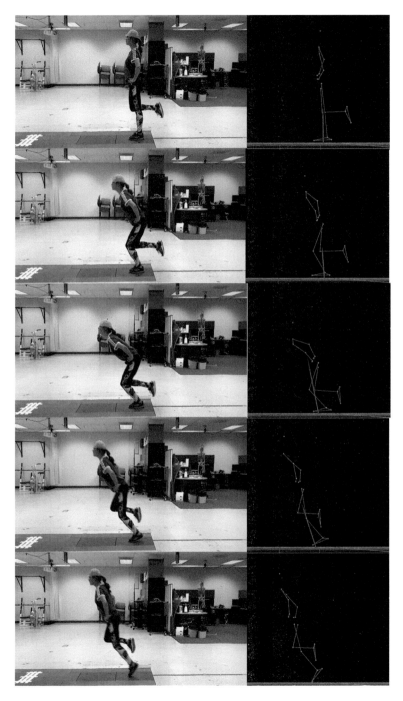

Figure 9.2 The magnitudes and directions of force vectors as shown by the red vectors during a forward jump.

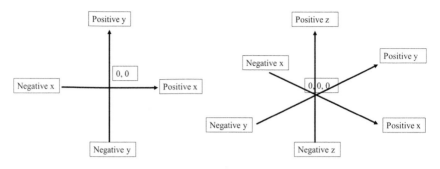

Figure 9.3 Two-dimensional (left) and three-dimensional (right) Cartesian coordinate systems.

Summary

In this chapter, we introduce the definition of biomechanics and provide examples of the application of biomechanics in sports training and injury prevention. We have discussed the basic definitions of linear and angular motion, kinematics, and kinetics, and compared and contrasted the similarities and differences between scalars and vectors and between two-dimensional and three-dimensional motion.

Questions for reflection

- Develop a biomechanical model of the maximal running speed in sprinting.
- Give other examples of linear vs. angular motion, kinematics vs. kinetics, and scalar vs. vectors.
- Find a video that shows the approach, takeoff, and flight of a high jump. Does high jump motion mainly occur in a two-dimensional or three-dimensional space? Please describe the movement directions in the approach, takeoff, and flight phases.

References

Chow, J. W., & Knudson, D. V. (2011). Use of deterministic models in sports and exercise biomechanics research. *Sports Biomechanics*, *10*(3), 219–233.

Hamill, J., Knutzen, K., & Derrick, T. (2015). *Biomechanical basis of human movement* (4th ed.). Philadelphia, PA: Wolters Kluwer.

Hatze, H. (1974). Letter: The meaning of the term "biomechanics". *Journal of Biomechanics*, *7*(2), 189–190.

10 Linear kinematics

Outcomes

- Defining linear position, displacement, velocity, and acceleration.
- Explaining the procedure of using a regular camera to capture linear position and calculate linear velocities and acceleration.
- Applying the projectile motion equations to understand possible optimal release angles in sports events.

Linear position, displacement, velocity, and acceleration

The variables used to describe linear kinematics include linear positions, displacements, velocities, and acceleration (Hamill et al., 2015). Below are the definitions of linear displacement, linear velocity, and linear acceleration.

Linear Displacement = Final Linear Position – Starting Linear Position

Linear Velocity = Linear Displacement/Time

Linear Acceleration = (Final Linear Velocity – Starting Linear Velocity)/Time

Position is the location of an object in space. A two-dimensional position can be described by the x and y locations, while a three-dimensional position includes anterior-posterior, left-right, and vertical locations. Displacement is the change in positions from the start to the end. Jump height is a displacement as it is the difference between the standing vertical position and the maximal vertical position in a jump. Velocity is the change in positions with respect to time. Velocities can be instantaneous velocities or average velocities. For an athlete who completes 100 meters in 10 seconds, the average velocity is 10 meters/second. However, it does not mean the velocity is constant. The velocity during the first 10 meters is typically slower than the velocity during the last 10 meters because the athlete starts from rest and needs time to develop velocities. Acceleration is the change in velocities with respect to time. Positions, displacements, velocities, and acceleration can be positive, zero, or negative. For a sprinter who decelerates after passing the finishing line, the velocity of the sprinter is still forward, but the acceleration is backward to slow down the forward velocity to come to a stop.

DOI: 10.4324/9781003331964-13

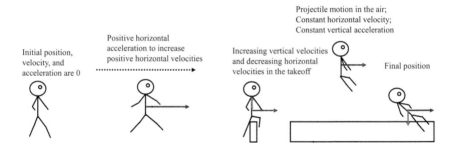

Figure 10.1 Changes in positions, velocities, and acceleration in the long jump.

In the long jump (Figure 10.1), the performance is the displacement between the takeoff board and the athlete's final position in the horizontal directions. If an individual can step on the takeoff board, he/she will have a good takeoff position. The horizontal velocity at the takeoff and the takeoff angle are determinants of the displacement in the air. To achieve a fast velocity at takeoff, the individual needs to accelerate from a velocity of 0 at the starting position in the early phase and maintain a fast velocity in the later phase of the approach.

In cyclic movements such as swimming, running, and cross-country skiing, linear velocities can be quantified for each cycle. Increased linear velocities can be caused by increased displacement or decreased time for each cycle. An analysis of elite swimmers showed that increased displacement per stroke accounted for faster velocities in certain events, while decreased time per stroke was more important in other events (Craig et al., 1985). An eight-week training increased novice cross-country skiers' cycle displacement and maintained the same cycle time, and resulted in increased cycle velocities in the poling and sliding phases (Li et al., 2021).

Quantification of positions

Many methods can be used to capture the position of an object. One convenient method is to use a regular camera to record a video at a specific sampling frequency. A picture can be treated as a two-dimensional Cartesian coordinate with the left bottom corner as the origin, the bottom line as the positive x, and the left line as the positive y. As such, all x and y positions in the picture have zero or positive values. In addition, the numbers of pixels in the x and y directions provide units of measurement.

As shown in Figure 10.2, the picture has 1920 pixels in a row and 1080 pixels in a column for a resolution of 1920*1080. Based on the scale of the pixels, the position of the center of the volleyball can be quantified using pixels. A calibration between real-world units (meters) and pixels can be performed by placing a 1-meter scale in the plane of motion. In this picture,

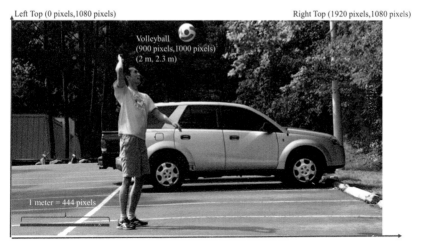

Figure 10.2 Capturing the position of an object using pixels and then converting it to meters using a calibration scale.

the calibration of a 1-meter scale resulted in 444 pixels, enabling the conversion from pixels to meters. When the motion is recorded as a video, multiple pictures are taken at a certain time interval. For example, Figure 10.3 shows the multiple pictures recorded in a video at a sampling frequency of 60 frames/second. As such, 60 pictures are taken in one second with a time interval of 1/60 second between two frames. As the position of the

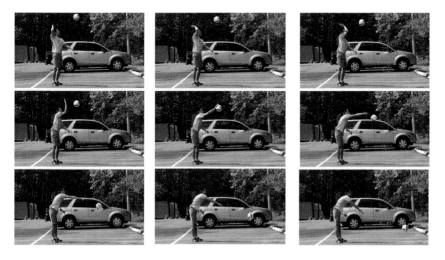

Figure 10.3 A video captures a series of pictures at a certain time interval. The velocity of the ball can be quantified based on the changes in positions and time.

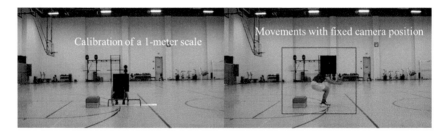

Figure 10.4 Sequences of calibration and motion capture of dynamic movements.

volleyball can be quantified in each frame, the velocities of the volleyball can be calculated as the changes in positions divided by the changes in time. Once the velocities are calculated for each frame, the acceleration of the volleyball can be quantified using the same steps.

The common procedure is to place a calibration scale in the plane of motion prior to the dynamic movement (Figure 10.4). The calibration scale is then removed, and the dynamic motion will be recorded. If the camera position is not moved, the conversion between pixels and meters will not change. However, three requirements need to be met for 2D motion capture using a regular camera: 1. The movement of the object is mostly in a single plane. 2. The camera is placed perpendicular to the movement plane to capture the movement plane. 3. The calibration scale is positioned in the movement plane.

The use of a single camera has been commonly used to quantify linear locations, distances, and velocities. For example, one study studies the relationship between the medial movement of the knee in a landing task and the risk of anterior cruciate ligament injuries in elite female handball and football athletes (Nilstad et al., 2023). With multiple cameras, 3D motion can be constructed with a 3D calibration tool and more complicated calculations (Dai et al., 2020).

Projectile motion

The projective motion involves horizontal displacement, horizontal velocity, and vertical velocity. Their definitions are provided below.

$$\text{Horizontal Displacement} = (V_x * \sqrt{V_y * V_y + 2gh} + V_x * V_y)/g$$
$$\text{Horizontal Velocity} = V_x = V_r * \cos(\theta)$$
$$\text{Vertical Velocity} = V_y = V_r * \sin(\theta)$$

In a special situation when the release height and landing height are the same, the variables involved in projectile motion are:

$$h = 0$$
$$\text{Time to Peak Height} = Vy/g$$
$$\text{Total flight time} = 2 * Vy/g$$
$$\text{Horizontal Displacement} = 2 * Vy * Vx/g$$

The horizontal displacement in projectile motion is determined by the release velocity (Vr), the release angle (Θ), the difference between the release height and landing height at the release (h), and gravity (g, about 9.8 m/s^2). The release velocity and release angle also determine the horizontal velocity (Vx) and vertical velocity (Vy). Increases in Vx, Vy, and h and a decrease in g will increase the horizontal displacement. When an object is projected into the air with negligible air resistance, gravity is the only force acting on the object. Therefore, the horizontal velocity is constant, and the horizontal acceleration is zero. The vertical velocity is up initially and reaches zero when the object is at its peak. Then, the vertical velocity is down before the object contacts the ground. The vertical acceleration is constant gravity. When the release height and landing height are the same, h is 0, and several simplified equations can be used. Overall, the vertical velocity determines how long the object will stay in flight, while the horizontal velocity will determine how far the object will travel during the flight time.

Release velocity is developed by an individual within a certain joint range of motion. An increase in strength and power can help increase release velocities: h is related to the release height and can help explain the advantages of taller individuals in throwing activities, and g is similar on Earth, but you may expect further displacement when you throw an object on a different planet with less gravity.

When the release height equals landing height with a constant release velocity, the optimal release angle to reach the furthest distance is 45 degrees. This optimal angle can be tested by releasing an arrow from a bow. If the deformation of the band is the same, the release velocity of the object will be constant. However, the actual release angle can significantly deviate from 45 degrees in human movements. For example, the takeoff angle in the long jump is about 20 degrees in elite male athletes, suggesting the horizontal velocity (~9 m/s) is much greater than the vertical velocity (~3 m/s) (Hay et al., 1986). The reason behind this deviation from 45 degrees is that long jumpers must spend more time in the takeoff if they want to increase the vertical velocity to increase the takeoff angle. However, the increase in takeoff time will decrease the horizontal velocity, so the overall takeoff velocity will decrease. The tradeoff between takeoff velocity and takeoff angle makes long jumpers favor keeping a high takeoff velocity rather than increasing the takeoff angle. As such, a constant release velocity at various release angles cannot be assumed for many throwing and jumping activities. The application of this equation is not limited to throwing with maximal effort but also throwing for accuracy. Infinite combinations of horizontal and vertical velocities can be used to reach the same displacement. A basketball shot can be made with a faster release velocity and a greater release angle or a slower release velocity with a smaller release angle. When a player performs a jump shot over an opponent, the player is likely to release the ball at a greater angle to avoid the opponent while still making the shot (Rojas et al., 2000).

Summary

In this chapter, we have defined linear position, displacement, velocity, and acceleration. We have described how to use a regular camera to capture linear positions. Linear velocities and acceleration can be calculated based on the changes in linear positions and time. Then, we have discussed the application of the projectile motion equations to understand the contributing factors to the horizontal distances in throwing activities. Different from machines, human bodies cannot change each projectile-motion factor independently.

Questions for reflection

- A running back started from standing and increased his speed to run forward (forward as the positive direction). His running speed slowed down because a defender pushed him backward. He finally stopped running because two more defenders tackled him. Please describe how the positions, velocities, and acceleration change from the start to the stop for this running back.
- A marker was placed on an individual's hip to capture a student's jump height. The vertical position of the marker at standing was 100 pixels. The maximum vertical position of the marker during jumping was 150 pixels. There were 200 pixels between the two points of a 1-meter calibration scale. What was the jump height in meters?
- The motion of a baseball was recorded at a sampling frequency of 60 frames/second. The position of the baseball at release was (1 m, 1 m). The position of the baseball after six frames was (4 m, 0.95 m). What was the average velocity of the baseball in the horizontal direction?
- A student releases a ball with a release velocity of 5 m/s at a release angle of 60 degrees. The release height is 2 m, and the landing height is 0 m. What is the horizontal travel distance of the ball ($g = 9.8$ m/s^2)?
- An object is released with a release velocity of 10 m/s at a release angle of 30 degrees. The release height and landing height are the same. What is the time for the object to reach its peak height? What is the total flight time? What is the horizontal travel distance? Will the ball travel further if the release angle is 45 degrees with the same release velocity ($g = 9.8$ m/s^2)?
- If a shot putter can release a shot with a constant release velocity, the optimal release angle will be about 42 degrees since the release height is slightly higher than the landing height. However, the actual release angle in elite shot putters is around 35 degrees. Please provide potential

explanations of why the actual release angle is smaller than the theoretical optimal release angle.

- The flight phase of a long jumper is a projectile motion. How can a long jumper increase his/her horizontal distance in flight based on the equation: Horizontal Displacement = $(Vx * \sqrt{Vy * Vy + 2gh} + Vx * Vy)/g$? As a coach, how can you use a regular camera to quantify these important parameters?

References

Craig, A. B. J., Skehan, P. L., Pawelczyk, J. A., & Boomer, W. L. (1985). Velocity, stroke rate, and distance per stroke during elite swimming competition. *Medicine and Science in Sports and Exercise*, *17*(6), 625–634.

Dai, B., Layer, J. S., Hinshaw, T. J., Cook, R. F., & Dufek, J. S. (2020). Kinematic analyses of parkour landings from as high as 2.7 meters. *Journal of Human Kinetics*, *31*, 15–28.

Hamill, J., Knutzen, K., & Derrick, T. (2015). *Biomechanical basis of human movement* (4th ed.). Philadelphia, PA: Wolters Kluwer.

Hay, J. G., Miller, J. A., & Canterna, R. W. (1986). The techniques of elite male long jumpers. *Journal of Biomechanics*, *19*(10), 855–866.

Li, J., Gao, B., Dai, B., Zhu, Q., Li, L., & Li, R. (2021). The effects of eight-week sports-specific training on the kinematics of double-pole techniques in novice cross-country skiers. Paper presented at the International Society of Biomechanics in Sports, Vol. 39: Iss. 1, Article 27.

Nilstad, A., Petushek, E., Mok, K., Bahr, R., & Krosshaug, T. (2023). Kiss goodbye to the 'kissing knees': No association between frontal plane inward knee motion and risk of future non-contact ACL injury in elite female athletes. *Sports Biomechanics*, *22*(1), 65–79.

Rojas, F. J., Cepero, M., Ona, A., & Gutierrez, M. (2000). Kinematic adjustments in the basketball jump shot against an opponent. *Ergonomics*, *43*(10), 1651–1660.

11 Angular kinematics

Outcomes

- Explaining and providing examples of segment and joint angles.
- Comparing the definitions of angular kinematics to linear kinematics.
- Applying a regular camera to capture and analyze segment and joint angles.
- Evaluating the relationships between linear kinematics and angular kinematics.

Segment angles and joint angles

A segment (absolute) angle is defined as the angle between the segment and the horizontal or vertical axis (Hamill et al., 2015). A joint (relative) angle is defined as the angle between two segments (Hamill et al., 2015). For example, the trunk segment angle is the angle between the trunk and the horizontal axis (Figure 11.1). The hip joint angle is the angle between the trunk and thigh segments. Joint angles are often the external angle formed by two segments so that the joint angle is 0 when the person is in the upright standing position. Segment and joint angles are often used to describe and modify movements. For example, athletes are often instructed to keep the trunk as straight as possible and lower the thigh to a parallel position in the back squat. The straight trunk and parallel thigh refer to segment angles. When a basketball player is instructed to bend hips and knees more while dribbling the ball, the instruction is related to joint angles.

Angular position, displacement, velocity, and acceleration

The variables used to describe angular kinematics include angular positions, displacements, velocities, and acceleration (Hamill et al., 2015). Their definitions and equations are provided below.

$$\text{Angular Displacement} = \text{Final Angular Position} - \text{Starting Angular Position}$$
$$\text{Angular Velocity} = \text{Angular Displacement/Time}$$
$$\text{Angular Acceleration} = (\text{Final Angular Velocity} - \text{Starting Angular Velocity})/\text{Time}$$

Angular positions, velocities, and acceleration are used to describe angular kinematics. Angles can be measured using degrees or radians. A circle is 360

DOI: 10.4324/9781003331964-14

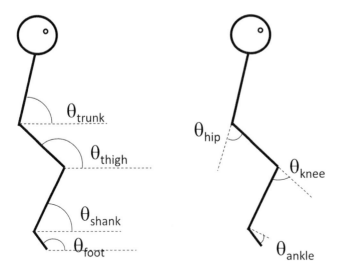

Figure 11.1 Lower extremity segment (left) and joint angles (right).

measured in degrees and 2*pi measured in radians. As such, 1degree is approximately 0.01745 radian, and 1radian is approximately 57.296 degrees.

The direction of angular motion can be described as clockwise or counterclockwise around a rotational axis, with the counterclockwise direction being defined as the positive direction. Most human motion involves segments rotating around joints, so angular kinematics are essential in describing body movements. Running can be analyzed as the center of the body moves in linear motion while different joints move in angular motion. A two-dimensional rotation involves joints rotating in a single plane. For example, knee flexion motion occurs in the sagittal plane, while shoulder abduction motion happens in the frontal plane. A three-dimensional rotation consists of rotations in three planes, such as knee flexion-extension in the sagittal plane, adduction-abduction in the frontal plane, and internal-external rotation in the transverse plane. The calculation of angular velocities from angular positions is like linear kinematics. Once the angles are captured with a certain sampling frequency, the angular velocities can be calculated as the changes in angular positions divided by the change in time.

In a forward-lunge exercise, as the person squats downward, the hip and knee move into greater flexion with flexion velocities (Figure 11.2), and the ankle moves into greater dorsiflexion with dorsiflexion velocities. When the person moves upward, the hip and knee decrease their flexion with extension velocities, and the ankle decreases its dorsiflexion with plantarflexion velocities. These sagittal-plane movements can be quantified using a single camera placed on the side of the person. Meanwhile, knee abduction is typically discouraged in this exercise, and this frontal-plane angle can be assessed with

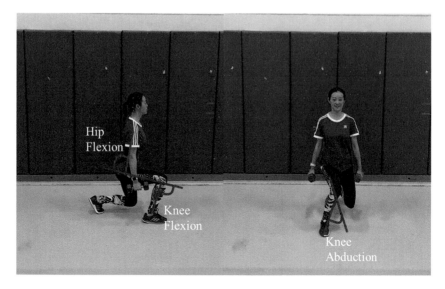

Figure 11.2 Hip flexion, knee flexion, and knee abduction in a forward-lunge exercise.

a camera placed in front of the person (Figure 11.2). Individuals typically land with decreased hip and knee flexion angles with a single leg compared with double legs due to the decreased single-leg strength (Donohue et al., 2015). When a person performs a squat with a front load (front squat), it can help decrease the flexion of the trunk (Gorsic et al., 2020).

Quantification of segment angles and joint angles

As mentioned in linear kinematics, the position of a joint can be captured using a regular camera. These positions can be further used to calculate segment and joint angles. Segment angles can be calculated using the arctangent function based on the differences in x and y between the two joints. Segment angles can then be used to calculate joint angles. Below is an example of calculating trunk and thigh segment angles and hip joint angles based on the positions of the shoulder, hip, and knee joints (Figure 11.3). The first step is to apply the arctangent function to the ratio of the differences in the y and x directions to calculate the segment angles. Then the joint angle can be calculated using the segment angles.

Angular to linear displacement

The definition and equation for angular to linear displacement are provided below.

Linear Displacement = Angular Displacement * Radius

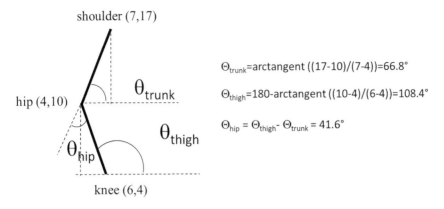

Figure 11.3 An example of calculating the trunk and thigh segment angle and the hip joint angle.

Angular displacement needs to be measured in radians. Referring to the number of loops a student has run is not informative unless you know the linear distance of each loop, which is determined by the size (radius) of the loop.

In a shoulder abduction exercise, the linear displacement of the dumbbell is determined by the angular displacement of the shoulder and the distance between the dumbbell and the shoulder (the length of the arm). As such, with the same angular displacement, the linear displacement will be greater for individuals who have longer arms. Taller rowing athletes will have advantages in generating a longer stroke with the same joint range of motion (Figure 11.4). A study found that the average body height was over 190 cm for males and over 180 cm for females in Olympic open-class rowers (Kerr et al., 2007). On the other hand, an Olympic lifter's goal is to lift the weight over the head instead of a certain height, so having a smaller body height will require a less linear displacement of the weight and may be advantageous.

Angular to linear velocity

The definition and equation for angular to linear velocity are provided below.

Linear Velocity = Angular Velocity ∗ Radius

The unit of the angular velocity needs to be radians/second. The release velocity (linear velocity of the object) is important in increasing throwing displacement. However, the linear velocity of the object is developed through the angular motion of different body joints. Understanding the conversion from angular to linear motion is important for evaluating the performance outcomes resulting from joint angular motion.

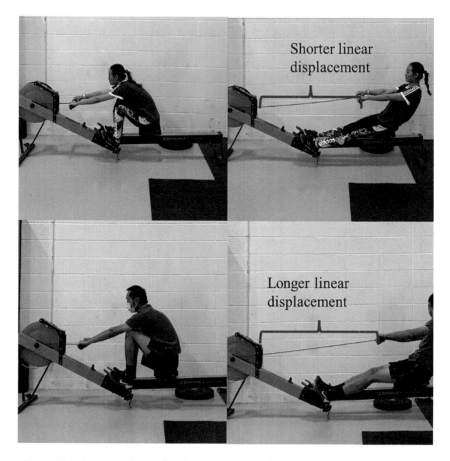

Figure 11.4 A longer linear displacement for a taller rower (bottom) with the same angular displacement.

To achieve a fast release velocity in throwing a ball, a student needs to develop fast angular velocities of different joints, including the wrist, elbow, shoulder, and trunk. In addition, a student should release the ball when the arm is close to fully extended to increase the radius of the rotation. Similarly, when a volleyball player tries to spike a ball with the maximal linear velocity of the hand. He/she should fully develop the angular velocities of the upper body and the arm and hit the ball with an extended arm (Figure 11.5). The use of a spear-thrower is another great example of increasing the radius between the rotational center of the angular motion to the object to increase throwing distances. Studies showed that different joint angles and angular velocities, such as elbow and shoulder rotation, contributed to the final velocity of the ball in baseball pitching (Crotin et al., 2022). In table tennis, the shakehand allows players to increase shoulder, elbow, and forearm

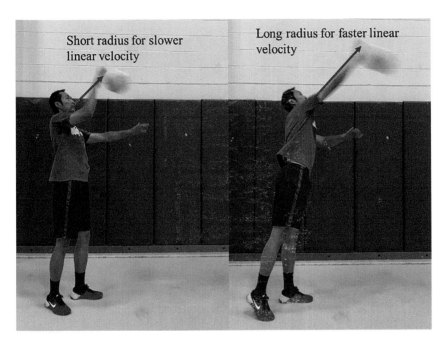

Figure 11.5 Hitting a volleyball with a bent or extended elbow and shoulder causes different radiuses.

motion because of the better alignment between the racket and the forearm to increase ball velocities for backhand strokes (Xia et al., 2020).

The signs of angular velocities and their contributions to the linear velocity should also be considered. A trunk flexion velocity instead of a trunk extension velocity will cause a forward linear velocity of the hand in throwing. In basketball shooting, the forward velocity of the ball is primarily produced by wrist flexion and elbow extension velocities, which also contribute to the upward velocities of the ball (Figure 11.6). The shoulder flexion velocities can contribute to the upward but backward velocities of the ball. As such, the elbow, which is further away from the ball (longer radius) compared to the wrist, appears to be a major contributor to both forward and upward velocities of the ball. The coordination of multiple joins results in the final release velocities of the ball. A study demonstrated that the angular velocities of the elbow increased most among shoulder, elbow, and wrist when the shooting distance increased from 2.8 m to 6.4 m (Okazaki & Rodacki, 2012). The major contributor may be targeted for intervention and training to improve performance.

Angular to linear acceleration

The definition and equation for angular to linear acceleration are provided below.

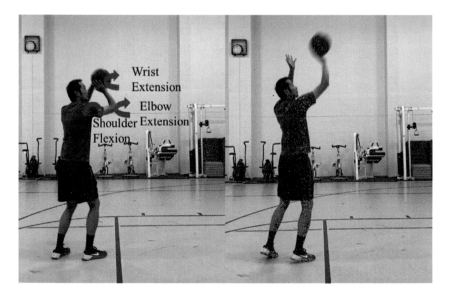

Figure 11.6 Different joint angular motion in basketball shooting.

Tangential Acceleration = Angular Acceleration $*$ Radius

Centripetal Acceleration = Angular Velocities^2 $*$ Radius

Centripetal Acceleration = Linear Velocities^2/Radius

The units need to be measured in radians. Two different equations can be used to calculate centripetal acceleration. Different from the equations to convert displacements and velocities, there are types of acceleration. The equation of tangential acceleration is like the equations for displacements and velocities. When there is a change in angular velocities, there will be angular acceleration to cause tangential acceleration. The direction of the tangential acceleration is perpendicular to the radial axis (Figure 11.7). However, even when the angular velocity is constant, the direction of the linear velocity is constantly changing. The centripetal acceleration, which points toward the rotational center, is to account for this constant change in the direction of the linear velocity. The forces to generate tangential acceleration and centripetal acceleration are called tangential forces and centripetal forces. The force is the product of acceleration and mass, which will be discussed in the linear kinetics section.

When a runner is sprinting around a turn, centripetal acceleration is needed to account for the change in the direction of linear velocities. This centripetal acceleration can be generated by the friction force. However, by leaning the body toward the center of the turn, this centripetal acceleration can be produced by the supporting force and body weight (Figure 11.8). Another example can be found in hammer throwing. When an athlete rotates to develop the

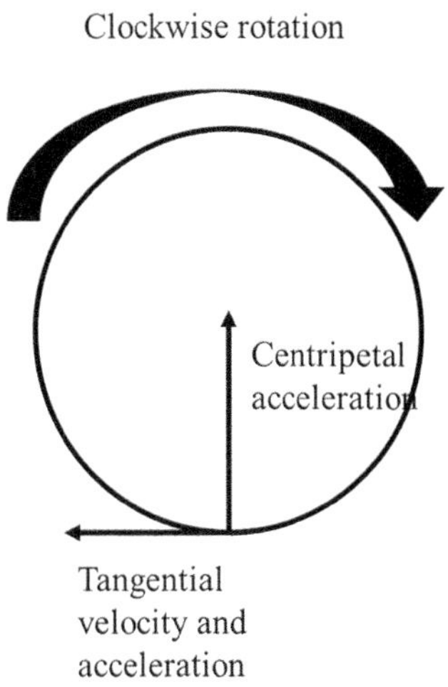

Clockwise rotation

Centripetal
acceleration

Tangential
velocity and
acceleration

Figure 11.7 Directions of the centripetal acceleration and tangential velocity and acceleration in a clockwise rotation.

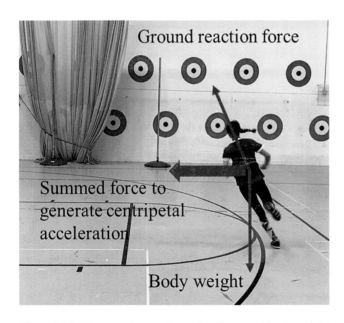

Ground reaction force

Summed force to generate centripetal acceleration

Body weight

Figure 11.8 The use of ground reaction force and body weight to generate centripetal forces and acceleration in a curve running.

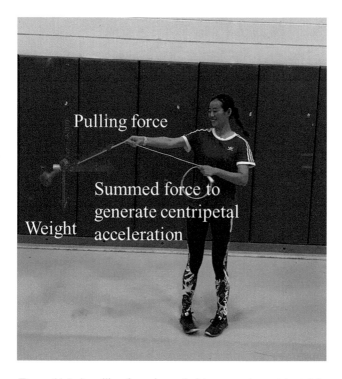

Figure 11.9 A pulling force is needed to generate centripetal forces and acceleration in a task like hammer throwing.

linear velocity of the hammer, the athlete needs to increase angular acceleration to develop angular velocity. However, the maintenance of a high angular velocity requires a centripetal acceleration to stabilize the hammer. The athletes need to pull the hammer toward the body to generate this centripetal acceleration (Figure 11.9). As the hammer is released after several rotations, too early developments of angular velocities will be detrimental to performance as the athlete may not have the strength to pull the hammer for stabilization. The ideal situation will be that the hammer reaches the highest angular velocity the athlete can control near the release of the hammer. A study showed that throwers could apply more than 2000 N of force to the cable in hammer throwing, and more than 90% of the force was used to generate centripetal acceleration to keep the hammer on track of a circle (Brice et al., 2011).

Summary

In this chapter, we have provided the definitions and examples of segment and joint angles. The definitions of angular displacement, velocities, and acceleration are similar to linear kinematics. We have explained the procedure to capture and analyze segment and joint angles and their applications in analyzing body movements. The equations to convert angular kinematics to linear kinematics have been defined and utilized to understand different motions.

Questions for reflection

- A club completes a wing in 0.5 seconds through a range of 180 degrees. What are the average angular velocities in degrees and radians per second?
- Please describe how the right ankle, knee, and hip joint angles change in a running stride (right heel strike to another right heel strike).
- Please calculate the thigh and shank segment angles and knee flexion angles based on the positions of the hip, knee, and ankle, as shown below.
- What is the linear distance if the angular displacement is 100 degrees, and the radius is 1 m? What is the tangential velocity if the angular velocity is 720 degrees/s, and the radius is 0.9 m?
- Point A is rotating counterclockwise. At this instance, point A is moving toward negative X. The angular velocity is 2 radians/s. The angular acceleration is 9 radians/s. The radius is 1 meter. Calculate tangential velocity, tangential acceleration, and centripetal acceleration. Draw the direction of these variables on the graph.
- Please provide examples of the conversion from angular kinematics to linear kinematics in exercise and sports activities and discuss how the changes in one variable may affect another.
- In softball batting, it is important to increase the linear velocity of the bat before hitting the ball. If an athlete can use a longer bat without decreasing the angular velocity of the bat, will it help increase the linear velocity of the bat? If an athlete must compromise the angular velocity of the bat when using a longer bat, will it help increase the linear velocity of the bat?
- When you make a turn in driving, centripetal acceleration is needed to keep the car in the circle. The centripetal acceleration is mainly provided by the friction force between the road and the tires. In snowy conditions, what are the things you can do to make sure that your car will stay on track during a turn?
- Please Go to https://www.kinovea.org/ to download the software for free. Take a picture when two people perform a body-weight parallel squat. Use the angle function of the software to quantify and compare the trunk angles and thigh angles at the lowest height between the two people.
- Anterior cruciate ligament (ACL) injuries are common in adolescent and young athletes. Research has suggested that athletes who tend to perform a landing task with a small knee flexion angle and a great knee abduction angle are more likely to suffer an ACL injury in the future. You are working as a sports scientist in the athletic department. At the beginning of a season, the athletic director has asked you to perform a baseline screening of the ACL injury risk for a group of basketball, soccer, and volleyball players. Please describe the equipment, procedure, and data analysis you plan to use for the screening.

References

Brice, S. M., Ness, K. F., & Rosemond, D. (2011). An analysis of the relationship between the linear hammer speed and the thrower applied forces during the hammer throw for male and female throwers. *Sports Biomechanics, 10*(3), 174–184.

Crotin, R. L., Slowik, J. S., Brewer, G., Cain, E. L. J., & Fleisig, G. S. (2022). Determinants of biomechanical efficiency in collegiate and professional baseball pitchers. *The American Journal of Sports Medicine, 50*(12), 3374–3380.

Donohue, M. R., Ellis, S. M., Heinbaugh, E. M., Stephenson, M. L., Zhu, Q., & Dai, B. (2015). Differences and correlations in knee and hip mechanics during single-leg landing, single-leg squat, double-leg landing, and double-leg squat tasks. *Research in Sports Medicine, 23*(4), 394–411.

Gorsic, M., Rochelle, L. E., Layer, J. S., Smith, D. T., Novak, D., & Dai, B. (2020). Biomechanical comparisons of back and front squats with a straight bar and four squats with a transformer bar. *Sports Biomechanics, 1*–16.

Hamill, J., Knutzen, K., & Derrick, T. (2015). *Biomechanical basis of human movement* (4th ed.). Philadelphia, PA: Wolters Kluwer.

Kerr, D. A., Ross, W. D., Norton, K., Hume, P., Kagawa, M., & Ackland, T. R. (2007). Olympic lightweight and open-class rowers possess distinctive physical and proportionality characteristics. *Journal of Sports Sciences, 25*(1), 43–53.

Okazaki, V. H. A., & Rodacki, A. L. F. (2012). Increased distance of shooting on basketball jump shot. *Journal of Sports Science & Medicine, 11*(2), 231–237.

Xia, R., Dai, B., Fu, W., Gu, N., & Wu, Y. (2020). Kinematic comparisons of the shakehand and penhold grips in table tennis forehand and backhand strokes when returning topspin and backspin balls. *Journal of Sports Science & Medicine, 19*(4), 637–644.

12　Linear kinetics

DOI: 10.4324/9781003331964-15

Outcomes

- Identifying the cause of motion and the basic components of forces.
- Explaining Newton's laws and how they can be applied to understand the cause of human movements.
- Introducing friction and air and fluid resistance equations.
- Applying the impulse and momentum equation to evaluate performance and injury risks.
- Defining linear work, energy, and power.

Force

Force (measured in Newtons) is the cause of linear motion. Force is a vector, and the three characteristics of a force are the magnitude, direction, and point of application (Hamill et al., 2015). For example, the distal point of application of the biceps is the forearm. The direction of the biceps force goes from the insertion (forearm) to the origin (shoulder) with a force to pull the forearm upward. The magnitude of the force is determined by the muscle strength and level of activation. In both deadlifts and back squats, the weight of the external load is pointing downward. The lifter applies force in the upward direction to overcome the weight of the external load. In a deadlift, the points of application are the hands, while the point of the application is the upper shoulder in back squats. Since force is a vector, a force can also be decomposed into the x and y directions as a velocity (Figure 12.1).

Mass and weight

The equation for mass and weight is listed below.

Weight = Mass * Gravity

Mass (kg) is a scaler that represents the resistance to linear motion. Mass does not have a direction and is not affected by gravity. Differently, weight is a vector and has a direction. On Earth, the weight points down to the center

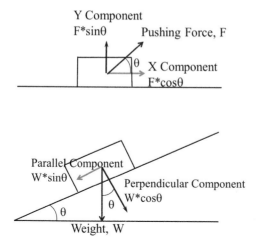

Figure 12.1 Examples of decomposing a force into two perpendicular directions.

of Earth and is about 9.8 times the mass. In addition, the further you are from the center of Earth, the less your weight will be. As such, your mass will be the same when you are standing at sea level compared to standing at a high altitude, but your weight will be less when you are standing at a high altitude. When the same person is standing on the moon, the mass will be the same, but the weight will only be about 1.6 times the mass.

Newton's first law

The equation for Newton's first law is listed below.

If $\sum F = 0$, then Linear Acceleration = 0.

$\sum F$ represents the sum of forces applied to the object in a specific direction. As such, if the total force applied to the object is zero in a direction, there will be no linear acceleration in that direction. The object will continue to be static or have a constant linear velocity. As previously mentioned, the horizontal velocity of an object is constant in the projectile motion when the air resistance is negligible because of no force acting on the object in the horizontal direction.

Newton's second law

The equation for Newton's second law is listed below.

$$\sum F = \text{Mass} * \text{Linear Acceleration}$$

When the sum of forces is not zero in a specific direction, it will generate linear acceleration in that direction. The only force acting on an object is the weight of the object in the projectile motion when air resistance is negligible.

As such, since weight is about 9.8 times the mass, the vertical acceleration of an object is about −9.8 m/s^2 in the projectile motion. In two-dimensional analyses, it is possible to have static analyses (zero acceleration) in one direction and dynamic analyses (non-zero acceleration) in another direction. The projectile motion is such an example.

When the goal is to develop the acceleration and velocities of an object with a constant mass, a greater absolute force will have advantages. For example, athletes in throwing events such as the shot put and discus throwing typically have large body sizes to develop greater absolute forces while the mass of the external object is constant (Figure 12.2). For offensive linemen in American football, their roles are to block and slow down the tacklesfrom the defensive players. Having a larger body size will help decrease the acceleration caused by the forces applied by the opponents.

Meanwhile, when the goal is to develop acceleration and velocities related to the body mass, the relative force (force/mass) is more important. Athletes such as high jumpers and long jumpers are typically smallerthan throwers. Javelin throwers are typically smallercompared to shot putters and discus throwers because they need to develop running velocities in the approach. In addition, wide receivers typically do not play through too much contact before catching a ball and are smallerthan linemen. The ratio between the

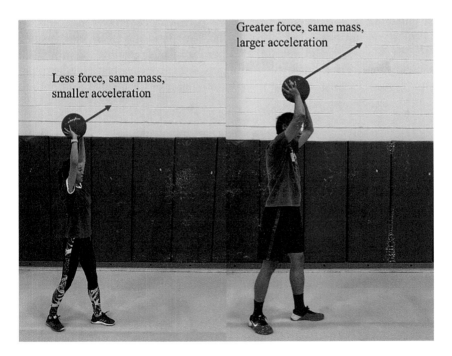

Figure 12.2 Larger body size is beneficial for generating acceleration when the external object has a constant mass.

force and body mass becomes critical in developing fast running speeds and jump heights. The relationship between forces, mass, and acceleration should be considered when we assess students' performance. A student/athlete who is good at throwing tasks does not necessarily demonstrate good jumping and running performance.

Newton's third law

The equation for Newton's third law is listed below.

Force a on b = −Force b on a

Newton's third law defines the action and reaction forces. Forces always act in pairs. The force object 1 applies to object 2 is the same as the force object 2 applied to object 1 in the opposite direction.

In a push-up exercise, the person extends the elbow and horizontally adducts the shoulder to push against the ground, so the person applies a downward force to the ground. Based on the law of action and reaction, the ground applies a force with the same magnitude in the opposite direction to the person to move the person up (Figure 12.3). This concept should also be considered between performance training and injury prevention. For example, a person is approaching to make a layup in basketball. A faster approaching speed may be advantageous to pass defenders for sports performance. However, as the last step of the layup is to slow down in the horizontal direction and generate vertical velocities, the leg must extend harder to push against the ground to generate more backward forces if the person approaches fast (Figure 12.4). While applying a great force to the external object or the ground is important

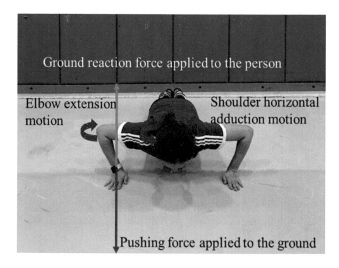

Figure 12.3 Action and reaction forces in a push-up exercise.

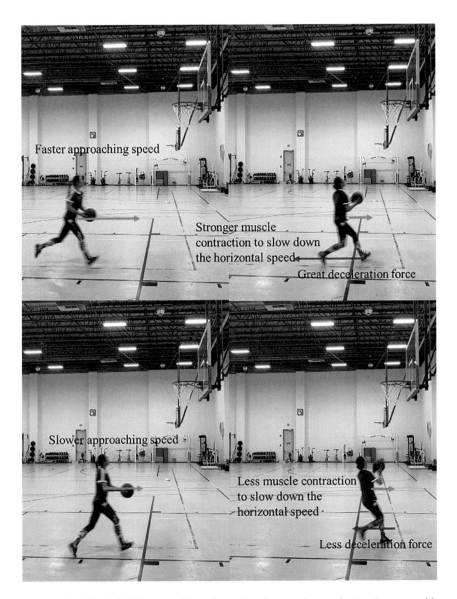

Figure 12.4 Basketball layup with a faster (top) or a slower (bottom) approaching speed.

for performance, the external object and ground will also impose loading on the body to increase injury risk. A study showed that the force applied to the leg increased while the jumping and cutting speeds increased (Dai et al., 2019). As such, beginners should avoid certain techniques used by elite athletes, which are likely to impose excessive loading on the body. Another example is helmet-to-helmet contact in American football. Sometimes you may see that the player who initiates the contact also experiences a concussion because the forces between the two helmets are the same. Meanwhile, you are more likely to see that the player who is targeted suffers a concussion because the targeted play is typically not as well prepared for the collision and will have less head stability than the player who initiates the contact, but it is not due to a greater force applied to the targeted player.

Surface friction

The equation for surface friction is listed below.

Friction Force = Normal Force $*$ Coefficient of Friction

Surface friction is defined as the force caused by the interface of two surfaces in contact with each other and can be categorized into static, sliding, and rolling friction forces determined by the compression and roughness of two surfaces (Hamill et al., 2015). Static friction is the friction force between two stationary objects, and the maximum static friction force is the maximum friction force to resist motion before movement occurs (Hamill et al., 2015). For example, when you are pushing a very heavy table, the table may not move, as your pushing force is counterbalanced by the static friction force between the table and the ground. Sliding and rolling friction forces are kinetic friction forces thatoppose relative linear and angular motion between two objects (Hamill et al., 2015). When a football player is running with a sled, there is a sliding friction force between the sled and the surface to increase the training load. The friction forces applied to moving wheelchairs and cars are rolling friction forces.

Friction can occur between the foot and the ground, between two bones, between the body and the air, and between the ball and the court. For example, a greater friction force exists between the tennis ball and the clay surface, resulting in slower ball velocities after the bounce compared to the grass surface. Soccer cleats can increase the friction between the shoe and the grass to increase an athlete's ability to decelerate and accelerate. Friction always opposes the relative motion between the two surfaces. Normal force is the compression force that's perpendicular to the two surfaces. When a person is standing on a flat surface, the weight is pointing down and perpendicular to the surface. However, when a person stands on a ramp, only a part of the weight (the cosine component) is perpendicular to the surface. Coefficients of friction are determined by the roughness and moving speeds between the two surfaces. The static coefficient of friction when an object is not moving is greater than the kinetic coefficient of friction when an object is moving. When you are pushing a desk on the ground, you may find it is harder to overcome the friction force to initiate the motion but easier to continue the motion once the object starts to move. The coefficients of rolling friction are much smaller than the coefficient of sliding friction. Pushing a wheelchair when it is not locked is much easier compared to when it is locked due to the smaller coefficient of friction.

Friction not only slows down an object but also causes acceleration. For example, the motion of your foot is to move forward relative to the ground at the heel contact of running. Hence, the friction force has a backward direction, acting to slow down the runner. However, the motion of your foot is to move backward relative to the ground during the push-off of running. Then the friction force acts forward to accelerate the runner (Figure 12.5). Consequently, running involves a constant phase of decelerating and acceleration due to the change in the direction of friction forces. The anterior and posterior forces collected by a force platform clearly showed that the force

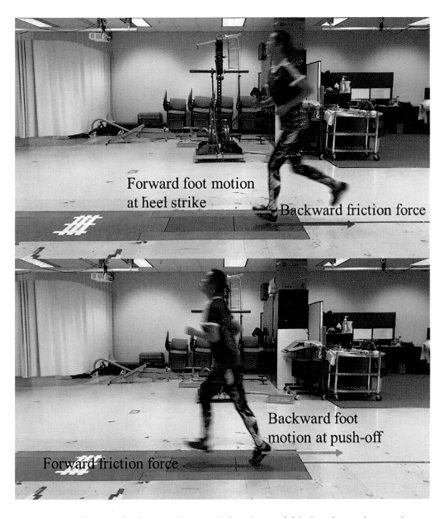

Figure 12.5 Changes in foot motion and directions of friction forces in running.

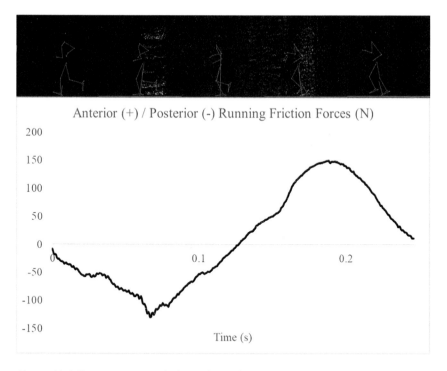

Figure 12.6 Force vectors and plots of anterior/posterior forces during running.

was acting backward during the early stance phase and then changed its direction to forward during the late stance phase (Figure 12.6). As previously mentioned, an offensive lineman prefers to have a large mass to have more resistance to acceleration. In the meantime, an increased weight will also have a greater normal force to increase the friction between the player and the ground to further decrease the acceleration resulting from the opponents. The coefficient of friction can be modified by changing surfaces and shoes. For example, artificial turfs tend to induce higher friction forces compared to natural grasses. The higher friction may allow athletes to perform accelerating and decelerating tasks more quickly. However, due to the law of force action and reaction, the high friction forces of the artificial turfs may also be associated with increased lower extremity loading and injury risk.

Maximum achievable incline method

The static coefficient of friction can be quantified using a simple method called the maximum achievable include method (Hsu et al., 2015). When the incline angle is increased to a point, the stational object placed on the surface will start to slide. The tangent of this critical angle when the object starts to slide is the static coefficient of friction (Figure 12.7). For example, a basketball coach was interested in the coefficient of static friction between new

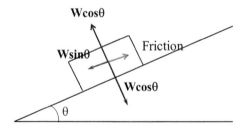
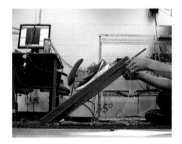

Wsinθ=Friction=Wcosθ*Coefficient of Friction

Coefficient of friction= Wcosθ / Wsinθ =tanθ

Coefficient of friction=tan35°=0.7

Figure 12.7 Measuring the coefficient of static friction using the maximum achievable incline method.

shoes and a floor surface. The coach placed one shoe on the surface with the same material as the floor and slowly raised the surface. The coach stopped raising the surface when the shoe started to slide and measured the angle between the surface and the horizontal direction to be 35 degrees. The coefficient of static friction was calculated to be 0.7 (tangent of 35 degrees). A previous study used this method to quantify the static coefficients of friction of swing dance shoes and tennis shoes and found greater coefficients of friction in swing dance shoes with a rubber bottom and tennis shoes compared to swing dance with a leather bottom. In addition, the leather-bottom shoes resulted in decreased knee loading during a swing dance rotation (Perala et al., 2018).

Air and fluid resistance

The equation for air and fluid resistance is listed below.

$$\text{Drag force} = 0.5 * \text{ air and fluid density} * \text{movement velocity}^2 * \text{cross-sectional area} * \text{drag coefficient}$$

The most common air and fluid resistance is the drag force, which is positively related to the density of the air or fluid, the relative velocity between the object and the air and fluid, the cross-sectional area of the object, and the drag coefficient (Hamill et al., 2015; Seifert et al., 2011). The drag forces can be further broken down into the skin friction drag and form drag (Hamill et al., 2015). The skin friction drag is caused by the contact between the air or fluid and the object. The friction drag is bound to the boundary layer flow between the skin and the air or fluid and can be categorized as laminar or turbulent (Figure 12.8). A laminar boundary layer with minimal exchanges of air or water between layers results in less friction drag compared to a

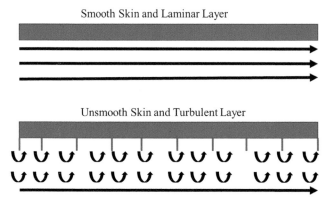

Figure 12.8 Laminar and turbulent layers.

turbulent boundary layer. The form drag is caused by the pressure difference between the front and the back of the object and is the most dominating component of the drag force in swimming (Figure 12.9). The form drag is not only affected by the frontal area of the object but also the shape of the object. When the air or water is connected at the front and back of the object, the air and water flow in the opposite direction of the movements (e.g., swimming and cycling directions) without disruption. This creates similar pressure at the front and back of the object and results in less form drag. When the air or fluid is not connected, the disruption will create higher pressure at the front and low pressure at the back of the object to resist the movement. Another way to conceptualize the form drag is through Newton's law of action and reaction. When the object is streamlined, the air or fluid flows smoothly from the front to the back without significant external forces applied to the air or

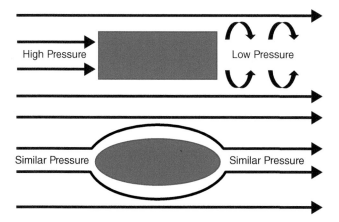

Figure 12.9 Object shape and form drag between the front and the back of the object.

fluid to disrupt the flow. When the object is not streamlined, the air or fluid will be slowed down by external forces. Meanwhile, the air and fluid apply an opposite force to the moving object to slow down the object's movements.

The density of air can be affected by the altitude of the location, as higher altitudes have less air density. As such, one may expect fast baseball throwing velocities and better speed skating performance at a higher altitude due to the decreased drag force. For cyclists and swimmers, wearing smooth hats and clothes will help create laminar layers and decrease the skin friction drag. Cyclists, speed skaters, and downhill skiers bend their knees and hips throughout the race to decrease the cross-sectional area to lower form drag (Figure 12.10). For swimmers, the deviation from a streamlined body will increase the cross-sectional area and decrease the smoothness of water flow to create form drag. Swimmers need to try to keep the head, spine, hips, and legs in a straight line that is parallel to the water surface to minimize form drag while swimming through the water (Figure 12.11). Not only in the up and down direction, but swimmers also need to minimize unnecessary side-to-side movements to optimize the streamlining of the body.

However, air resistance does not always decrease athletes' performance. The propulsive force in swimming also comes from the drag force between the relative motion of the body and water. For example, most of the propulsion forces in freestyle swimming come from the motion of the arms. As the arm is moving and pushing the water backward, the water is applying a reaction force to the arm to move the body forward. While the arm is moving forward in the air, the friction force applied by the air is minimal. Meanwhile, when the leg is kicking the water backward, the water is applying a reaction force to the legs to swim forward. But when the leg is kicking the water forward, the water applies a drag force to the legs to slow down the swimmer. In discus

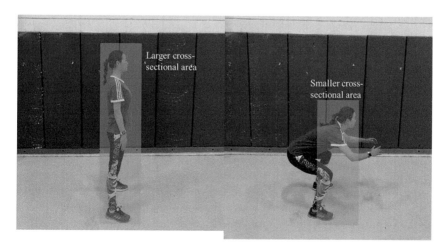

Figure 12.10 Different cross-sectional areas in the forward direction by changing body posture.

Non-streamlined Body   Streamlined Body

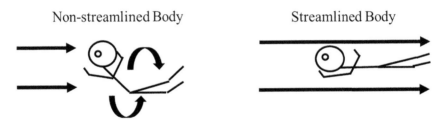

Figure 12.11 A streamlined body (right) will have less form drag in swimming.

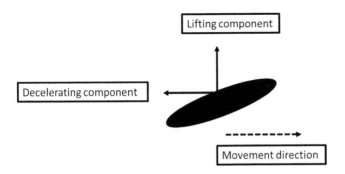

Figure 12.12 Lifting and decelerating components of the dragging force when a discus is in the air.

throwing, some athletes' throwing distances are longer than the theoretical distance based on their release velocities and heights. This is because a part of the drag force is acting to lift the discus under certain discus orientation and travel directions (Figure 12.12). When the gain in flight time due to the lifting overcomes the loss in velocities due to the deceleration component, the travel distance is increased.

Wave drag

Wave drag is another drag that is caused by the waves of water when the swimmer is gliding directly below the water surface (Figure 12.13) (Seifert et al., 2011). Wave drag depends on the speed of the swimmer, the length of the swimmer, and the depth of the swimming. The faster the speed, the shorter the swimmer, and the closer to the water surface, the greater the wave drags. The hull speed is a speed where the wavelength equals the swimmer's length. Swimmers must spend more energy climbing over the wave to further increase speed when the swimmer's speed reaches the hull speed.

When the swimmer is swimming further below the water surface at the start or a turn, there is less wave drag as the swimmer is not directly below the

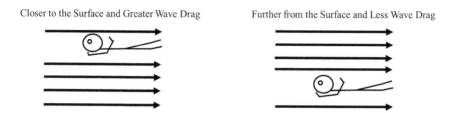

Closer to the Surface and Greater Wave Drag   Further from the Surface and Less Wave Drag

Figure 12.13 Gliding closer to the water surface will have greater wave drag.

water surface. A longer boat or a taller swimmer can move at a faster speed to reach the hull speed before experiencing significant wave drag compared to a shorter boat or shorter swimmer.

Magnus effects

The Magnus effect is observed that when a spinning object is moving through the air or fluid, its trajectory will deviate from a straight line due to the pressure differences applied to the different sides of the object (Hamill et al., 2015). As an object is moving forward and spinning in one direction, one side of the object is spinning in the same direction as the incoming air or fluid, while the other side of the object is spinning in the opposite direction to the incoming air or fluid. The side with the same directions will have a fast speed of the air or fluid and lower pressure. The side in the opposite direction will have a slow speed of the air or fluid and higher pressure. This difference in pressure will change the trajectory of the object (Figure 12.14).

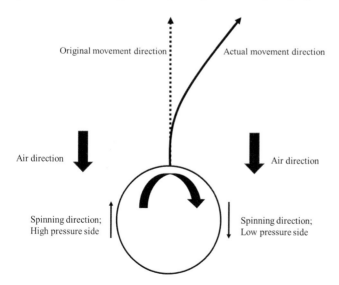

Figure 12.14 Demonstration of the Magnus effects for a spinning ball.

The application of the Magnus effect is very common in sports. Spinning the ball around the vertical axis will create a deviation in the left and right directions and is the mechanism that creates curveballs in soccer kicking and baseball throwing. Spinning the ball around the left-right axis will cause the ball to drop quickly or stay in the air for long. For example, a topspin volleyball involves the ball spinning around the left-right axis forward. As such, the top of the ball experiences greater pressure than the bottom of the ball, resulting in a quick drop of the ball.

Linear impulse and momentum

The equation for linear impulse and momentum is listed below.

$$Force * Time = Change\ in(Mass * Linear\ Velocity)$$

When a force is applied to an object for a period, it will change its linear velocity. Impulse is the product of force and time. Momentum is defined as mass times velocity (Hamill et al., 2015). For example, if a 10 N force is applied to a 2 kg mass for 3 seconds, it will cause a change of 15 m/s of linear velocities of the object. A great force with a long time of application is the strategy to develop a fast velocity.

In throwing, an increased time of application typically involves a greater range of motion. The linear velocity of the wrist is primarily developed through the elbow joint in Figure 12.15, so the hip, shoulder, and elbow linear velocities are small and make minimal contributions to the wrist velocity. On the other hand, the linear velocity of the wrist is developed through the trunk, shoulder, and elbow joints in Figure 12.16, so there are progressive developments of linear velocities of the shoulder, elbow, and wrist to reach a fast final wrist velocity. Elite baseball throwers have an excellent shoulder internal-external range of motion to increase the time they can apply force to the baseball. In jumping activities, individuals typically squat down first to gain a large range of motion for the upward jumping motion. Athletes also tend to use a proximal to

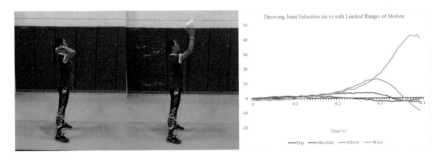

Figure 12.15 Throwing with small joint ranges of motion decreases the time to generate an impulse.

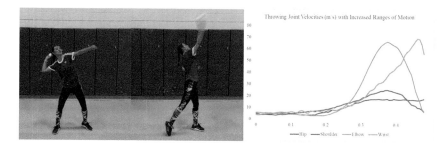

Figure 12.16 Throwing with large joint ranges of motion increases the time to generate an impulse.

distal control strategy to increase the duration. Instead of starting the motion of all contributing joints at the same time, the proximal joints (trunk) typically rotate and reach peak velocities first, followed by the distal joints (wrist in throwing and ankle in jumping, Figure 12.16).

However, there is a limit to when a large range of motion and an increased time can contribute to the increased impulse because the total force output may decrease when the range of motion is too large. Having a person start a squat jump from the deepest position may not increase jump heights as the deepest position may not make a significant contribution to the upward velocity. The impulse and momentum equation can also be applied from a different perspective. When the goal is to stop an object's velocity, a longer time will decrease the peak force that is needed. For example, when an individual lands from a jump, he/she can use a "soft" landing technique by increasing knee and hip flexion to prolong the time to stop the downward velocity (Figure 12.17). Due to the increased time, the peak force acting on the individuals will decrease to minimize the risk of acute injuries. Similar principles can be applied to falling on concrete

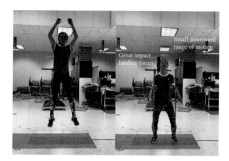 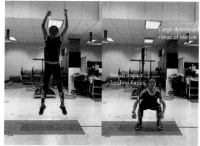

Figure 12.17 A stiff landing with small joint ranges of motion increases the impact landing forces, and a soft landing with large joint ranges of motion decreases the impact landing forces.

compared to on a gymnastic mat, which will result in a longer time and a less peak force to decelerate the body. Previous studies showed that both soft landing and safe falling techniques could reduce the impact forces (Dai et al., 2015; Li et al., 2020). Elite Parkour athletes utilize the whole-body range of motion and rolling forward techniques to land from as high as 2.7 meters (Dai et al., 2020). When a baseball player tries to catch a fastball, the player can move the hand backward in the catching motion to increase the time to slow down the ball. The peak force acting on the hand will then be decreased.

Conservation of momentum

The equation for conservation of momentum is listed below.

Sum of (Momentum Before) = Sum of(Momentum After)

Conservation of momentum defines that the momentum of a system of multiple objects will be constant if the external force applied to the system is zero. This equation is an extension of the impulse-momentum equation. For example, small pieces of a static object will travel in different directions in an explosion as the sum of the momentum of all the small pieces will be zero.

When two football players collide in the air, each player applies a force to the other player in the horizontal direction with opposite directions. The external force acting on these two players is zero in the horizontal direction. After the collision, the two players will travel in the direction of the player who has more momentum before the collision. For example, if player 1 (100 kg)'s velocity is 5 m/s and player 2 (60 kg)'s velocity is 6 m/s, both players will travel in the same direction as player 1, who has a greater momentum (500 kg*m/s vs. 360 kg*m/s) before the collision.

Coefficient of restitution

The equation for the coefficient of restitution is listed below.

$$e = -\frac{V2f - V1f}{V2i - V1i}$$

For situations when one object is bouncing on a stationary object, the equation is:

$$e = \sqrt{\frac{Hbounce}{Hdrop}}$$

e is the coefficient of restitution. V1i, V1f, V2i, and V2f are the initial and final velocities of the two objects. Bounce is the height of the bounce, and

Hdrop is the height of the drop. The coefficient of restitution of two colliding objects is a value representing the ratio of speeds after and before an impact (Inaba et al., 2017). The coefficient of restitution is commonly used in sports to define the characteristics of collision among sports equipment. For example, the coefficients of restitution are about 0.85 for tennis racquets and 0.83 for basketball.

Before the collision, Ball 1 is moving towards the right with a speed of 3 m/s. Ball 2 is moving towards the left with a speed of 1 m/s. After the collision, Ball 1 is moving towards the right with a speed of 1 m/s. Ball 2 is moving towards the right with a speed of 2 m/s. The coefficient of restitution is calculated a–(2 − 1)/(−1 − 3) = 0.25. A golf ball was dropped from a height of 1 m to the ground. After the collision, the golf ball bounced back to a height of 0.6 m. The COR between the golf ball and the ground is calculated as $\sqrt{0.6/1}$. =0.77.

Linear work and energy

The equations for linear work and energy are listed below.

$$
\begin{aligned}
\text{Linear Work} &= \text{Force} * \text{Linear Displacement} * \\
&\quad \text{Cos(angle between the force and displacement)} \\
\text{Work} &= \text{Change in (Energy)} \\
\text{Translational Kinetic Energy} &= \tfrac{1}{2} * \text{Mass} * \text{Linear Velocity}^2 \\
\text{Potential Energy} &= \text{Mass} * \text{Gravity} * \text{Height} \\
\text{Strain Energy} &= \tfrac{1}{2} * \text{stiffness} * \text{deformation}^2
\end{aligned}
$$

Linear work is defined as the product of force and displacement in the same direction, and energy is defined as the capacity to do work (Hamill et al., 2015). When the force and displacement are in the same direction, the angle is 0, and cos (angle) is 1. When the force and displacement are in the opposite direction, the angle is 180, and the cos(angle) is −1, indicating negative work. When a football player is running with a sled forward, the player is performing positive work on the sled to increase its velocity. When a skier moves down a hill, the friction force performs negative work on the skier to slow down the skier.

Translational kinetic energy is defined as the energy resulting from linear motion and is determined by the mass and velocity of the object (Hamill et al., 2015). A rugby player with great mass and a fast running speed will have great kinetic energy. Potential energy is defined as the capacity to do work due to the object's position and is determined by the mass and height of the object (Hamill et al., 2015). As a skier moves down from the top to the bottom of the mountain, the potential energy decreases and kinetic energy increases. Mechanical energy is the sum of kinetic and potential energy. Strain energy is defined as the energy caused by the object's deformation and released as elastic energy and is determined by the stiffness and deformation of the materials (Hamill et al., 2015). In the pole vault, the athlete's kinetic energy transfers to the strain energy of the pole, which is later transferred to the potential energy of the athlete to cross over the bar.

In the descending phase of back squats, the body is doing negative work because the upward force and downward movement are in the opposite direction. On the other hand, the body is doing positive work in the ascending phase. When you perform work on an object, it will change its energy. For example, when you lift a dumbbell up, you perform positive work on the dumbbell to increase its potential energy. When you are pitching a baseball, your body performs work to increase the kinetic energy of the ball. Energy can also transfer from one form to another. When a skier slides down a hill, most of the potential energy is transferred to kinetic energy, while a part of the energy is lost due to the negative work done by the friction force (Figure 12.18). Muscle tendons can serve to store strain energy. At the toe touch of sprinting, the Achilles tendon is stretched to store strain energy. At the push-off, the Achilles tendon is shortened to release the strain energy. When an individual falls on a mat, the kinetic energy of the person is transferred to the deformation (strain energy) of the mat. The pole vault is another great example of the transfer of different energy. The pole vaulter starts from the rest with zero kinetic and potential energy. The athlete performs positive work to run to increase the kinetic energy in the horizontal direction. This kinetic energy is then transferred to strain energy when the pole is bent. When the pole is straightening, the strain energy is converted back to the athlete's kinetic energy and potential energy.

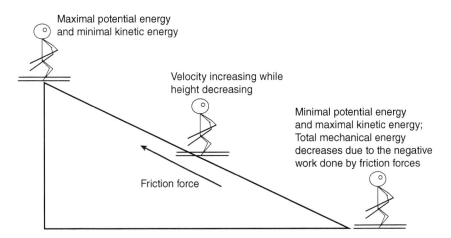

Figure 12.18 Changes in potential and kinetic energy and negative work done by the friction force in the downhill ski.

Linear power

The equations for linear power are listed below.

Power = Change in(Work)/Change in(Time)
Power = Force * Velocity

Units of power are Watts. Power is defined as the changes in work relative to time (Hamill et al., 2015). Work is defined as force times displacement, so power can also be defined as the product of force and velocity. Power can be positive or negative, depending on whether the force and velocity point in the same or opposite direction. Power is an important factor in assessing movements and designing training. While strength is defined as the maximal force a person can produce during a certain task, power is affected by both forces and velocities. Due to the muscle force-velocity relationship, the maximal muscle force decreases when the muscle contracting velocity increases. Therefore, the peak power typically occurs at a force level much less than the peak force.

The peak power you produce in throwing an empty bar might be greater than the peak power in a maximal bench press. You may have observed that some individuals can perform back squats with a significant number of loads relative to body weight, but they can not jump very high. This is due to the back squat being a slow movement to evaluate peak force production, while the vertical jump test was a power test determined by the takeoff velocity. Lifting or jumping with less external loads will generate greater velocity with smaller forces (Figure 12.19). Lifting or jumping with more external loads will result in slower velocities with greater forces. The optimal load to maximize power could be task-specific and individual-specific. A previous study found that holding a dumbbell of 10% of body weight increased peak jumping power compared to holding a barbell or wearing a vest because of the arm

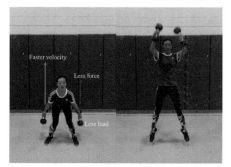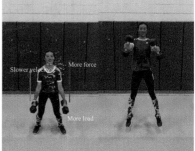

Figure 12.19 Jumping with less external loads has faster velocities but less force (left) and jumping with more external loads has slower velocities but more forces.

movement in increasing power (Bordelon et al., 2022). In addition, performing push-ups with 5% or 10% of body weight in a weighted vest increased peak force but decreased peak velocities and showed similar peak power compared to push-ups without extra weights (Hinshaw et al., 2018). For many movements such as throwing, jumping, and running, during which velocity is the determining factor, power will play an important role and has implications for training specificity.

Summary

In this chapter, we have discussed force as the cause of linear motion and the three basic components of forces. We explain Newton's laws I, II, and II and their application in understanding the cause of motion. We have introduced surface friction and air and fluid resistance to understand the role of friction in locomotion and how air and fluid resistance might affect swimming and other sports performance. We have emphasized the impulse and momentum equation to evaluate the relationships between performance and injury risks and defined linear work, energy, and power.

Questions for reflection

- Describe the three characteristics of the patellar tendon muscle force.
- A 1000 kg car starts to roll down a very icy road (ignoring the friction force) with a 30-degree incline (g = −9.8 m/s^2). How much force must be applied in the direction of the road to stop the car?
- Will your mass and weight change when you are standing in Columbus, Ohio (elevation: 270 m) compared to standing in Laramie, Wyoming (2,200 m)?
- Discuss other events in which the absolute force or relative force might be more important than the other.
- Two forces are applied to an object. Force 1 is (10 N, 20 N), and force 2 is (20 N, −30N). The mass of the object is 10 kg. What is the acceleration in the X and Y directions?
- Please give other examples of force action-reaction.
- A football player's mass is 100 kg. The coefficient of friction between the player and the grass is 1. What is the friction force between the player and the grass? How could the player increase this friction force?
- Based on the Surface Friction equation (Force = Normal Force * Coefficient of Friction), why is it hard to push a shopping cart full of groceries compared to an empty cart? Why is it harder to push the cart on grass compared to tiles? Why is it hard to start moving a full cart at the beginning and easy to maintain the speed once it starts to move?
- How do the relative motion between the foot and ground and the direction of friction force change during a single-leg side hopping task?
- Use the Maximum Achievable Incline Method to quantify and compare the coefficients of friction between two types of shoes and a surface.

- In several swimming styles, a swimmer must break the water surface at a distance no greater than 15 meters at starts and turns. From the perspective of skin, form, and wave drag, please explain why dolphin kicking will experience less drag compared to surface swimming.
- Does a basketball shot typically involve a topspin or a backspin? How will the spin affect the trajectory of the ball?
- Please list other applications of impulse/momentums in exercises and sports.
- A 0.3 kg softball is traveling at a velocity of 70 m/s. If a force over 300 N can injure the hand, what is the shortest time it will take to catch the ball without injuring the hand? How can a player decrease the peak force based on the impulse/momentum relationship?
- An 80 kg player is moving at a horizontal speed of 10 m/s and collides with a stationary 70 kg player in the air. After the collision, these two players move at the same horizontal speed. What is the horizontal velocity of the two players after the collision?
- For table tennis, the ball should bounce up about 25 cm when dropped from 30 cm onto a steel block. What is the coefficient of restitution between the ball and the block?
- A diver (mass = 70 kg) is 10 meters above the water. How much potential does she have? A diver (mass = 70 kg) hits the water after a dive from the 10 m tower with a velocity of 14 m/s. How much linear kinetic energy does she possess when she hits the water? A muscle tendon with a stiffness of 70,000 N/m is stretched by 0.01 m. How much strain energy does it have?
- A bench press exercise could be performed with a load of 50 kg with a movement velocity of 0.2 m/s or with a load of 20 kg with a movement velocity of 0.6 m/s. Which load and movement velocity would result in greater movement power?
- Should the training for lower extremity strength and power be different? Why?
- An individual exerts a horizontal force of 100 N at a horizontal velocity of 2 m/s. What is the power generated? If the power is generated constantly for 5 seconds, what is the work generated?
- For a person who has just started downhill skiing, what will be effective strategies to maintain a low speed so that the injury risk is minimized? Please explain from the perspective of work and energy.

References

Bordelon, N. M., Jones, D. H., Sweeney, K. M., Davis, D. J., Critchley, M. L., Rochelle, L. E., ... Dai, B. (2022). Optimal load magnitude and placement for peak power production in a vertical jump: A segmental contribution analysis. *Journal of Strength and Conditioning Research*, *36*(4), 911–919.

Dai, B., Garrett, W. E., Gross, M. T., Padua, D. A., Queen, R. M., & Yu, B. (2015). The effects of 2 landing techniques on knee kinematics, kinetics, and performance during stop-jump and side-cutting tasks. *The American Journal of Sports Medicine*, *43*(2), 466–474.

Dai, B., Garrett, W. E., Gross, M. T., Padua, D. A., Queen, R. M., & Yu, B. (2019). The effect of performance demands on lower extremity biomechanics during landing and cutting tasks. *Journal of Sport and Health Science, 8*(3), 228–234.

Dai, B., Layer, J. S., Hinshaw, T. J., Cook, R. F., & Dufek, J. S. (2020). Kinematic analyses of parkour landings from as high as 2.7 meters. *Journal of Human Kinetics, 31*(72), 15–28.

Hamill, J., Knutzen, K., & Derrick, T. (2015). *Biomechanical basis of human movement* (4th ed.). Philadelphia, PA: Wolters Kluwer.

Hinshaw, T. J., Stephenson, M. L., Sha, Z., & Dai, B. (2018). Effect of external loading on force and power production during plyometric push-ups. *Journal of Strength and Conditioning Research, 32*(4), 1099–1108.

Hsu, J., Li, Y., Dutta, T., & Fernie, G. (2015). Assessing the performance of winter footwear using a new maximum achievable incline method. *Applied Ergonomics, 50*(5), 218–225.

Inaba, Y., Tamaki, S., Ikebukuro, H., Yamada, K., Ozaki, H., & Yoshida, K. (2017). Effect of changing table tennis ball material from celluloid to plastic on the post-collision ball trajectory. *Journal of Human Kinetics, 30*(55), 29–38.

Li, L., Baur, M., Baldwin, K., Kuehn, T., Zhu, Q., Herman, D., & Dai, B. (2020). Falling as a strategy to decrease knee loading during landings: Implications for ACL injury prevention. *Journal of Biomechanics, 26109*(109), 109906.

Perala, H. D., Wilson, M. A., & Dai, B. (2018). The effect of footwear on free moments during a rotational movement in country swing dance. *Journal of Dance Medicine & Science: Official Publication of the International Association for Dance Medicine & Science, 22*(2), 84–90.

Seifert, L., Chollet, D., & Mujika, I. (Eds.). (2011). *World book of swimming: From science to performance*. Hauppauge, NY: Nova Science Publishers.

13 Angular kinetics

Outcomes

- Understand the center of mass calculation and how the center of mass interacts with the base of support.
- Explain the two components of torque and how the direction of a force might affect its moment arm; Define different types of levers and how they may affect mechanical advantages.
- Define moment of inertia as the resistance to angular motion.
- Evaluate how the change of moment of inertia might affect angular velocity with a constant angular momentum.
- Quantify rotational kinetic energy and angular work and power.

Center of mass and center of gravity

The equations for center of mass are listed below.

$$COM = \frac{\sum_{i=1}^{n} Mi * Xi}{\sum_{i=1}^{n} Mi}$$

$$COM = \frac{\sum_{i=1}^{n} Mi * Yi}{\sum_{i=1}^{n} Yi}$$

Center of mass (COM) is a virtual point about which an object's mass is evenly distributed (Hamill et al., 2015). In the two equations, the nominator includes the sum of the product of the mass and position of each segment. The denominator is the sum of the mass of each segment. The center of mass of an individual is not a fixed point because each segment can change its position. The center of mass is around the pelvis when an individual stands in the anatomical position. The center of mass can move outside of the body if there is external support, such as holding a cane and leaning on a wall.

To calculate the center of mass of the three objects: Object 1 (5 kg)'s location is (2, 3). Object 2 (3 kg)'s location is (2,1). Object 3 (2 kg)'s location is (4, 4).

DOI: 10.4324/9781003331964-16

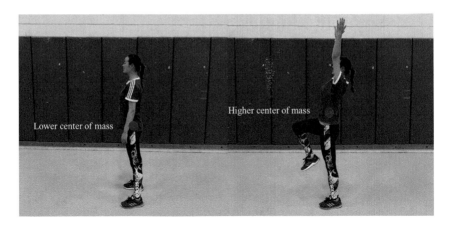

Figure 13.1 A posture like the high-jump takeoff increases the center of mass position in the vertical direction.

X direction:

m1 * x1 + m2 * x2 + m3 * x3
5 * 2 + 3 * 2 + 2 * 4 = 24 kg * m
m1 + m2 + m3
5 + 3 + 2 = 10
X center of mass = 24/10 = 2.4 m

Similarly, Y center of mass can be calculated as 26/10 = 2.6 m

A high center of mass will be preferable at takeoff in the high jump. The high takeoff center of mass is achieved by raising both arms above the head as well as lifting the non-jumping leg at the takeoff (Figure 13.1). In addition, when a high jumper clears the bar, the Fosbury-Flop technique with a good back arch may allow the athlete to pass the bar when the center of mass is below the bar to gain extra bar height. When an individual is performing a double-leg squat, the center of mass is typically located in the middle of the two feet, with equal weights being distributed between the two legs (Figure 13.2). However, individuals following a major lower extremity injury tend to shift their center of mass toward the non-injured leg to decrease the weight distributed on the injured leg. Studies have found that patients following anterior cruciate ligament injuries shifted their bodies to the non-injured side to unload the injured side (Song et al., 2021, 2023).

Base of support

The base of support is the area formed by the outside edge of the body parts and other tools in contact with the ground (Hamill et al., 2015). When a person is standing with a single leg, the base of support is the size of the

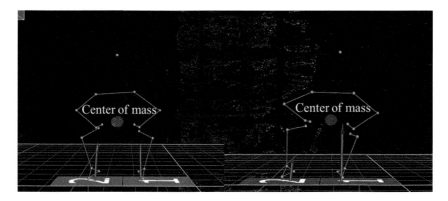

Figure 13.2 Symmetric and asymmetric squats with different center of mass locations.

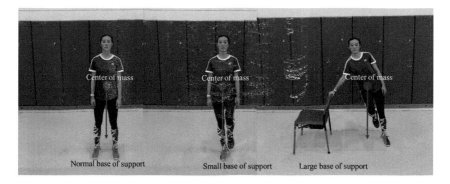

Figure 13.3 Different sizes of bases of support.

support foot (Figure 13.3). For a double-leg stance, the base of support includes the two feet and the inside areas between the two feet.

The relationship between the center of mass and the base of support is important for maintaining balance. For static balance, the center of mass needs to be aligned with the base of support. A single-leg stance is harder due to its decreased base of support compared to a double-leg stance. Commonly used static balance tests include single-leg balance and tandem stance with or without eyes open (Dai et al., 2012).

Torque and moment arm

The equation for torque is listed below.

Torque = Force * Moment Arm

Torque (Nm) is the cause of angular motion. Moment arm is the perpendicular distance from the force line of action to the rotational center (Hamill et al., 2015). The torque of a force is largely determined by the direction and point of application of the force.

A seesaw may tilt to the person with less weight if the person sits further away from the center compared to the person with greater weight. When you are holding heavy objects, you will try to bring them as close to you as possible because it will decrease the distance from the weight of the object to your body joints. By holding the end of the wrench, you increase the moment arm of the force to generate a greater torque to rotate a bolt. The moment arm can also help analyze and develop training exercises. When someone is performing a biceps curl exercise at a slow speed, the most challenging position is when the forearm is in the parallel position, representing the greatest perpendicular distance from the weight to the elbow (Figure 13.4).

As shown in Figure 13.5, there are two torques applied to the lever. Since the lever is perpendicular to the forces, the moment arms will be 2 meters and

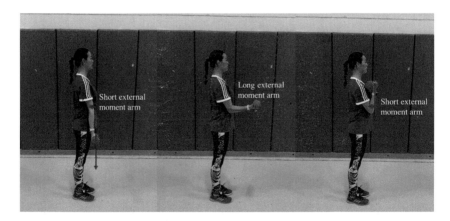

Figure 13.4 The moment arms between the load and elbow joint at different joint positions during a bicep curl exercise.

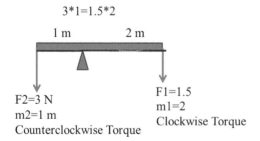

Figure 13.5 Static analyses of torques.

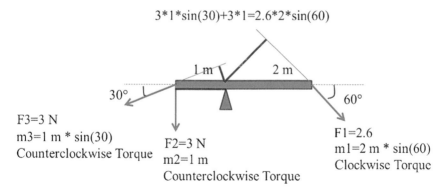

$$3*1*\sin(30)+3*1=2.6*2*\sin(60)$$

1 m   2 m

30°   60°

F3=3 N
m3=1 m * sin(30)
Counterclockwise Torque

F2=3 N
m2=1 m
Counterclockwise Torque

F1=2.6
m1=2 m * sin(60)
Clockwise Torque

Figure 13.6 Static analyses of torques.

1 meter for force 1 and force 2, respectively. Since force 2's moment arm is two times force 1's moment arm, its force is only half of force 2 to maintain a static position.

Figure 13.6 shows that the moment arm of the force can be different if the force is not applied in the perpendicular direction of the lever. In this case, the perpendicular distance needs to be drawn from the rotational center to the force line of action. Forces 1 and 3's moment arms are the sin components of the lengths of the lever. The sum of the clockwise torques equals the sum of the counterclockwise torques to maintain a static position.

Classes of levers

Based on the location of the effort force, resistance force, and fulcrum, a lever can be classified as a first-, second-, or third-class lever (Hamill et al., 2015). The first class has the fulcrum point between the effort and resistance force. Examples include seesaws and scissors (Figure 13.7). The second class has the resistance force between the effort force and the fulcrum. Examples include wheelbarrows and bottle openers (Figure 13.7). The third-class level has the effort force between the fulcrum and resistance force and is commonly

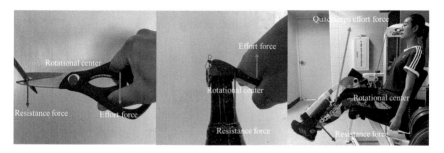

Figure 13.7 The first-, second-, or third-class levers.

observed in the human body, such as biceps curls and knee extension exercises (Figure 13.7). The third-class levels are more common in sports. When an athlete is holding a piece of equipment such as a javelin, a racket, or a bat, the weight (resistance force) of the equipment is acting at the distal location of the bone, while the muscle forces (effort force) are acting at the proximal location of the lever between the joint (fulcrum) and the resistance force.

Mechanical advantages

The ratio of the effort arm to the resistance arm is called the mechanical advantage (Hamill et al., 2015). When the mechanical advantage is 1, the lever simply redirects the applied force. A scale and a seesaw with an equal distance to each seat are such examples. When the mechanical advantage is greater than 1, the level acts to amplify force with a greater range of motion. The bottle opener in Figure 13.7 has a mechanical advantage greater than 1 as the effort force is applied further away from the rotational center compared to the resistance force. When the mechanical advantage is less than 1, the level acts to amplify the range of motion with greater forces. Human joints mostly have a mechanical advantage less than 1, meaning the muscles need to generate greater forces to move small external objects. As shown in Figure 13.7, the resistance force is applied further away from the knee joint compared to the quadriceps force, meaning a great muscle force is needed to lift a small amount of external load. The low back muscle may need to generate 1,800 N of force to lift a box that is 100 N. The compressive force acting on the low back discs could be greater than 10,000 N when elite athletes perform deadlifts (Cholewicki et al., 1991). This is due to the large moment arms from the external object to the low back joint along with a small moment arm from the low back extensors to the low back joint.

Internal and external forces, moment arms, and torques

Human muscles generate forces around joint centers to produce joint torques. For example, the biceps muscles pass around the center of the elbow to generate elbow flexion torques in the sagittal plane. The gluteus medius muscles pass around the hip joint to generate hip abduction torques in the frontal plane. These muscle forces, moment arms, and torques represent internal forces, moment arms, and torques. While muscle forces are generated to move external objects, the external objects will impose external forces and torques. For example, during a leg extension exercise (Figure 13.7), the quadriceps produce internal forces around the knee joint. The quadriceps act away from the knee joint with an internal moment arm, resulting in internal torques with a tendency to rotate the joint. Meanwhile, the external load is applied to the distal shank, representing the external force. This external force acts away from the knee joint with an external moment arm to impose external torques.

The relationships between internal and external torques help to understand the observation of many exercises. An individual typically can squat more loads with a half squat compared to a full squat. This is because the external

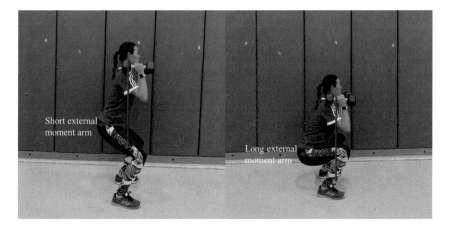

Figure 13.8 A lower squat depth increases the external moment arms from the loads to the hip joint.

moment arms of the external load will increase as the squat depth increases, making the external torques on the knee, hip, and low-back joints greater. However, the internal forces and moment arms associated with the low-back, hip, knee, and ankle extensors are not likely to change much as the squat depth changes. Therefore, the maximal load an individual can squat typically decreases with an increased squat depth (Figure 13.8).

Stability

Stability is the ability of an object to recover its original posture after its posture is perturbed by linear or angular acceleration (Hamill et al., 2015). The stability of human postures is largely affected by the center of mass location, base of support, and magnitude of the perturbation.

A person who stands straight will be more likely to fall after a pushing force is applied because the pushing force will have a longer moment arm to the foot, while the weight will have a shorter moment arm to the foot (Figure 13.9). The person will be more stable with a lower center of mass and a wider stance, which is commonly used when volleyball and basketball players play defense to maintain a stable position.

Moment of inertia and angular acceleration

The equations for moment of inertia and angular acceleration are listed below.

Angular Acceleration = Torque/Moment of Inertia
Moment of Inertia = Mass $*$ Radius of Gyration^2

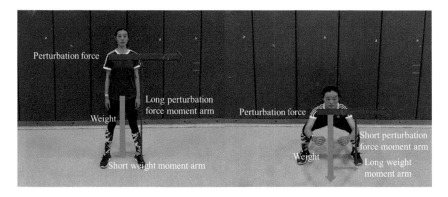

Figure 13.9 A lower center of mass and a wider stance increase the moment arm of the weight and decrease the moment arm of the perturbation force to increase the stability.

Torque is the cause of angular motion, while the moment of inertia is the resistance to angular motion. (Hamill et al., 2015) Angular acceleration is calculated as the torque being divided by the moment of inertia. Therefore, a great torque with a small moment of inertia will generate a great angular acceleration.

Moment of inertia is determined by the mass and the distribution of the mass around the rotational axis (Hamill et al., 2015). The radius of gyration is determined by the distribution of the mass, with the closer the mass to the rotational axis, the less the radius of gyration. Whole-body rotations can occur around the anterior-posterior, medial-lateral, and vertical axes, with the mass being the closest to the vertical axis (Figure 13.10). As such, the vertical axis has the least moment of inertia (resistance to rotation) and the fastest rotation in many movements. While the total mass of an object is

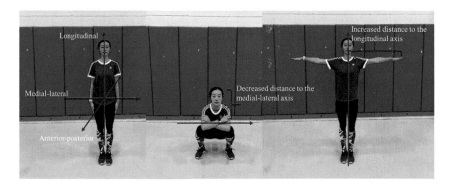

Figure 13.10 Three axes of rotation and modifying moments of inertia by changing body postures.

constant, the distance from each mass component to the rotational axis can be manipulated. For example, by bending the arms, trunk, and legs to reach a squat position, a person can decrease the distance from these segments to the medial-lateral axis to decrease the moment inertia.

Conservation of angular momentum

The equation for conservation of angular momentum is listed below.

Sum of(Moment of Inertia ∗ Angular Velocity Before)

  = Sum of(Moment of Inertia ∗ Angular Velocity After)

Like linear kinetics, the total angular momentum of a system is constant when the external torque acting on the system is zero (Hamill et al., 2015). When an individual is in the air with negatable air resistance, the only force acting on the individual is the force due to gravity. As gravity is acting on the center of mass, the external torque applied by the gravity around the center of mass is 0. Therefore, the conservation of angular momentum can be applied to projectile motion, such as diving, high jump, and long jump. With the same angular momentum, the posture in the middle of Figure 13.10 will demonstrate faster angular velocities around the medial-lateral axis compared to the posture on the left due to the decreased moment of inertia. Meanwhile, with the same angular momentum, the posture on the right will demonstrate slower angular velocities around the vertical axis compared to the posture on the left due to the increased moment of inertia.

Divers may change their body postures to decrease their moment of inertia to increase their angular velocity with the same angular momentum. First, the fastest rotation a diver can rotate is around the vertical axis (twists) since the vertical axis has less moment of inertia compared to the medial-lateral axis (somersaults). Second, for the rotations around the same axis, the number of rotations that can be achieved is different for different postures. For example, the straight posture has the greatest moment of inertia and, therefore, will have the least number of rotations with the same angular momentum. On the other hand, the tuck posture has the least moment of inertia and will result in the greatest number of rotations (Figure 13.11). Third, precise control of the timing of "open (increasing moment of inertia with slow rotation)" and "close (decreasing moment of inertia with fast rotation)" is critical in determining the close-to-vertical body posture when the diver enters the water. If the diver opens too early, the rotation will not be enough to reach a vertical body posture for water entry. If the diver opens too late, the rotation will be too much and pass a vertical body posture for water entry. Fourth, since the angular momentum is constant in the air, the takeoff phase before the flight phase is critical for generating the angular momentum. A diver needs to jump as high as possible to gain more flight time while generating enough angular

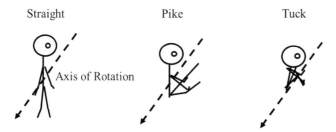

Figure 13.11 Straight (greatest moment of inertia around the medial-lateral axis), pike, and tuck (least moment of inertia) postures in diving.

momentum during the jumping phase so that the required number of rotations can be completed. Other examples include figure skaters and dancers who will bring their arms closer to their bodies to decrease their moment of inertia around the vertical axis to increase their angular velocity. Long jumpers will rotate their upper body clockwise while the lower body rotates counterclockwise to maintain the same angular momentum.

Angular work

The equation for angular work is listed below.

Angular Work = Torque * Angular Displacement

Like linear work, angular work is defined as the product of torque and angular displacement (Hamill et al., 2015). In a shoulder abduction exercise, the external load is moved in the vertical direction, and the linear work can be calculated as the product of the force and vertical displacement. In the meantime, the shoulder joint is performing angular work, which equals the shoulder joint torque times the shoulder angular displacement. Therefore, there are two ways to increase the shoulder joint work, with one being increasing external torque and the other one being increasing shoulder range of motion. While linear work is more relevant to the work done to the external object, angular work is directly related to the work the body has performed. The same linear work may involve different angular work performed by different joints. For example, lifting an object from the ground to the waist with straight legs (stoop lifting, Figure 13.12) primarily involved the low back performing the angular work. On the other hand, lifting an object with bent legs (squat lifting, Figure 13.12) involves greater contributions from the lower extremity work. The total angular work can also be greater for squat lifting compared to stoop lifting because a greater part of the body weight needs to be elevated in the lifting phase. As such, the squat lifting might be more protective for the low back but require greater work to be done for each lift.

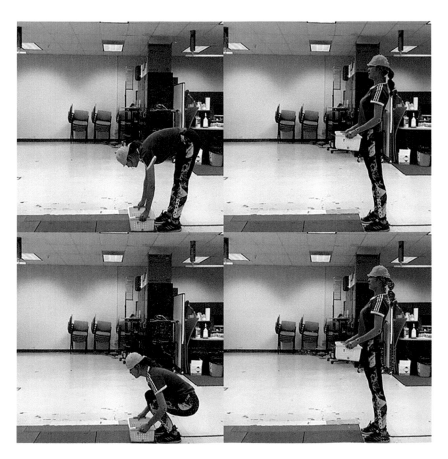

Figure 13.12 Stoop lifting (top) and squat lifting (bottom).

Change in angular momentum

The equation for change in angular momentum is listed below.

Torque * Time = Change in(Moment of Inertia * Angular Velocity)

As an extension of the conservation of momentum, a change in angular momentum will occur when there is an external torque acting on the object (Hamill et al., 2015). We have previously mentioned that the angular momentum of a diver is constant when the diver is in the air because there is no external torque acting on the diver. However, this constant angular momentum is generated through the external torque produced by the ground reaction force during the jumping phase before the diver leaves the platform. Again, it is essential for the diver to have a good jumping ability to generate a high angular momentum so that a fast angular velocity can be achieved in the

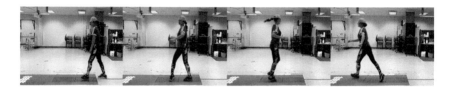

Figure 13.13 A rotational movement with the generation of angular momentum
during the double-leg stance phase and a decrease of angular
momentum during the single-leg stance phase.

flight phase. The same concept can be applied to dance movements such as
the pirouette, in which the dance's goal is to complete angular rotations
around one supporting leg. Before the rotation starts, the dancer pushes the
other leg to generate an external torque and rotates the trunk, arms, and legs
toward the rotational direction to generate a high angular momentum
(Figure 13.13). As shown in Figure 13.14, the force generated by the front-leg
force points to the right, while the force generated by the back-leg force

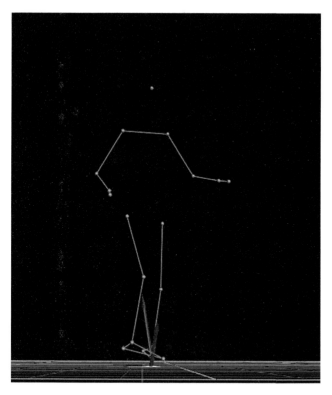

Figure 13.14 The front view of the rotational movement during the double-leg stance
phase.

points to the left. Both forces generate counterclockwise torques around the center of mass to increase the body's angular momentum during the pushing phase. After the angular rotation is initiated, the friction force between the dancer and the floor generates an opposite external torque to decrease the angular momentum and slow down the angular motion. Therefore, several factors, such as a high initial angular momentum, a small moment of inertia, and a small friction force between the dance and the floor, are important for achieving a high rotational speed.

Rotational kinetic energy

The equation for rotational kinetic energy is listed below.

$$\text{Rotational Kinetic Energy} = \frac{1}{2} * \text{Moment of Inertia} * \text{Angular Velocity}^2$$

In addition to linear kinetic energy, rotational kinetic energy is related to the angular velocity of an object (Hamill et al., 2015). For a bicycle wheel that is spinning without linear motion to the center, the linear kinetic energy is zero, but the rotational energy is non-zero due to the angular velocities. For two baseballs traveling at the same velocity, the baseball with greater rotational velocity will have a greater total kinetic energy.

Angular power

The equation for angular power is listed below.

$$\text{Angular Power} = \text{Torque} * \text{Angular Velocity}$$

As the definition of linear power, angular power is related to the magnitudes of torques and angular velocities (Hamill et al., 2015). When linear power is commonly used to assess whole-body power, angular power is used to determine joint power. When an individual is performing a leg extension exercise, which can be used to train kicking power for soccer players, we can expect a greater knee torque when the external load is heavy. On the other hand, a faster velocity will be observed when the external load is decreased. An optimal load between 0% and 100% of the maximal load is likely to maximize the knee joint power in training. Training with resistance bands is getting more and more popular among athletes. One advantage of this type of training is that individuals can perform a specific task, such as throwing, jumping, and kicking, with a lighter external load to maximize power.

Summary

This chapter describes the equations to calculate the center of mass, torque, and moment of inertia. The relationship between the center of mass and the base of support may affect stability. Different levers, including human bones, muscles, and joints, can be used to amplify forces or speeds and range of motion. The moment of inertia is related to the total mass as well as the distribution of the mass and acts to resist the generation of angular acceleration.

Questions for reflection

- Try to only stand on your left leg and reach both of your hands to your left as much as possible. What has happened to your right leg when you are reaching to your left? Why?
- Try to stand on a single leg and then stand on a single leg with your arms continuously moving to the left and right. Why is the second task harder to maintain a balance?
- What is the class of lever of a wheelbarrow? Is the mechanical advantage of a wheelbarrow greater, equal to, or less than one?
- The weights and moment arms of the dumbbell and right arm are shown in the figure below. Calculate the shoulder joint torque that is needed to maintain a static posture. If the shoulder torque is purely generated by the deltoid muscle, which has a moment arm of 0.05 m, what is the deltoid muscle force?
- For a 1-meter springboard dive with two somersaults around the medial-lateral axis, the straight posture will have a difficulty score of 2.6, while the pike and tuck postures have scores of 2.3 and 2.2. Why does the straight posture impose a greater difficulty?
- Low-back injuries commonly occur in workers who must perform many manual material-handling tasks such as lifting, carrying, and moving. Why does the lower back experience a significant amount of loading when a relatively small weight is lifted? What are the changes we can make to decrease the low-back loading during lifting tasks?
- Please discuss the changes in external moment arms associated with the load around the elbow and shoulder joints when bench presses are performed with a grip of one-shoulder-width apart or two-shoulder-width apart.
- Please discuss the changes in external moment arms associated with the load around the hip and knee joints when back squats are performed with a relatively straight or forward lean trunk.
- Please perform a curl-up exercise with your arms by your side or above your head. Which arm position is harder? Why?
- Please ask a friend to sit on a desk or chair. You will resist his/her lower leg when he/she is trying to extend the knee and move the lower leg forward as hard as possible. Try to hold his/her lower leg around the ankle or around the middle of the lower leg. Which holding location is harder for you to stop the forward motion of his/her lower leg? Why?
- The mass of a person is 100 kg. The mass of the thigh is 10% of the body mass. The radius of gyration of the thigh is 0.02 m^2. What is the moment of inertia of the thigh? If a torque of 10 Nm is applied to the thigh, what is the angular acceleration?

- The average height of elite female gymnasts is around five feet. How would a short height be advantageous in gymnastics? Please explain it from the perspective of the moment of inertia.
- The torque is 5 Nm. The angular displacement is 3.14 rad. The time of application is 0.5 seconds. What is angular work? What is an angular impulse?
- Moment of inertia is $0.5 \, \text{kg} \cdot \text{m}^2$. Angular velocity is 2 rad/s. What is angular momentum? What is rotational kinetic energy?
- Sitting on a rotating chair and asking a person to rotate the chair. Try to move your arms and thighs away from the chair and bring them closer to the chair. How do the angular velocities change when you are moving your arms and legs and why? Try to find a figure skating video that shows similar changes in angular velocities.
- Please watch a diving video that involves rotations around the medial-lateral and longitudinal axis. Which axis involved fast rotation? Why?
- An increased number of angular rotations in the flight will increase the difficulty score of the vault. What are the biomechanical concepts that can be applied to achieve an increased number of angular rotations?

References

Cholewicki, J., McGill, S. M., & Norman, R. W. (1991). Lumbar spine loads during the lifting of extremely heavy weights. *Medicine and Science in Sports and Exercise*, *23*(10), 1179–1186.

Dai, B., Ware, W. B., & Giuliani, C. A. (2012). A structural equation model relating physical function, pain, impaired mobility (IM), and falls in older adults. *Archives of Gerontology and Geriatrics*, *55*(3), 645–652.

Hamill, J., Knutzen, K., & Derrick, T. (2015). *Biomechanical basis of human movement* (4th ed.). Philadelphia, PA: Wolters Kluwer.

Song, Y., Li, L., Albrandt, E. E., Jensen, M. A., & Dai, B. (2021). Medial-lateral hip positions predicted kinetic asymmetries during double-leg squats in collegiate athletes following anterior cruciate ligament reconstruction. *Journal of Biomechanics*, *128*, 110787.

Song, Y., Li, L., Jensen, M. A., & Dai, B. (2023). Using trunk kinematics to predict kinetic asymmetries during double-leg jump-landings in collegiate athletes following anterior cruciate ligament reconstruction. *Gait & Posture*, *102*, 80–85.

Section 4

Observation, evaluation and diagnosis, and intervention

The integrated biomechanical model of qualitative skill analysis consists of four components: preparation, observation, diagnosis and evaluation, and intervention. We present preparation in Chapter 3. In this section, we will focus on the last three components: observation, evaluation and diagnosis, and intervention. Chapter 14 defines observation and discusses effective strategies for observation and how to conduct effective observations. Chapter 15 defines the third component of evaluation and diagnosis and discusses how to conduct evaluation and diagnosis based on biomechanical principles and prioritize errors for interventions. The final chapter (Chapter 16) presents the last component of intervention and discusses a variety of intervention methods to correct errors for better performance.

DOI: 10.4324/9781003331964-17

14 Observation

Outcomes

- Understand what observation is.
- Apply strategies to observe students' or athletes' performance for effective teaching or coaching.
- Apply steps to conduct effective observations.

Definition of observation

The second component of the Integrative Biomechanical Model of Qualitative Skill Analysis is observation. Observation is to use effective observational strategies to observe and record the performer's skill performance (Knudson & Morrison, 2002). The purpose of observation is to gather information about students' or athletes' skill performance for evaluation and diagnosis. Very often, teachers or coaches use an observational instrument to collect information for formal assessments. For informal assessments such as feedback, teachers or coaches do not use an observational instrument. They compare the observed performance with the ideal performance stored in their brain, and then immediately provide feedback to students or athletes for improvement. During observation, teachers or coaches only record the exact performance that students or athletes display during practices or game plays and any notes that will be useful for evaluation and diagnosis. Table 14.1 presents an example of an observation of soccer shooting skill using skill analysis observational sheet.

Strategies for effective observation

The data collected during observation is key to evaluation and diagnosis. Therefore, teachers or coaches must possess effective observational strategies. The following section will introduce eight effective observational strategies for teachers or coaches to consider during their observation.

Focus of observation

Prior to observation, teachers or coaches need to know what to focus on during observation. In general, teachers or coaches should focus on the

DOI: 10.4324/9781003331964-18

Table 14.1 Observational sheet for soccer shooting skill

Phase	Critical elements	Present? (yes/no)	Comments
Preparation	1 Feet shoulder width		
	2 Face target		
	3 Knees bent		
	4 Back straight		
	5 Eyes on target		
Execution	1 Approach to the ball		
	2 Elongated stride prior to planting foot beside the ball		
	3 Plant the non-kicking foot beside ball		
	4 Shift weight to non-kicking foot		
	5 Bring kicking foot backward with knee bent		
	6 Swing kicking foot forward straightening the knee		
	7 Square foot to ball		
	8 Make contact with ball		
Follow through	1 Kick through the ball		
	2 Land on kicking foot first then non-kicking foot		

biomechanically based critical elements to identify major errors in their students' or athletes' performance and then design interventions to fix those errors. However, based on the skill levels and experiences of students or athletes, teachers or coaches can have some flexibility in terms of what critical elements at which phase(s) to focus on. Beginning students or athletes will make numerous errors in their performance, which can be scattered in all three different phases. It is recommended that teachers or coaches focus on all the critical elements at all three phases to identify all errors, and then zoom in on major consistent errors in the following observation. Intermediate or advanced students or athletes will make very few errors. Teachers or coaches already know what those errors are. Therefore, teachers or coaches can mainly focus on those few errors during their observation.

Observational settings

What is the environment where practices occur? It can be an inside gym or an outside field. A major issue related to observation settings that teachers or coaches should pay close attention is distraction. If there are a lot of distractions during practices, students or athletes will lose their attention. This often leads to the occurrence of errors in their performance. Therefore, teachers or coaches should avoid conducting observations of students' or athletes' performance in any setting where there are a lot of distractions.

Athletes' or students' characteristics

Students or athletes vary in their skill levels and experiences. Beginning students or athletes will make more errors than those who are experienced and advanced. They typically miss several critical elements in a phase or even an entire phase of a skill. Their performance will change dramatically from one trial to the next trial. They may miss one critical element in one trial but perform correctly in the next trial. Therefore, during observations, teachers or coaches need to focus on identifying errors that beginning students or athletes consistently make in their performance. Those consistent errors are what teachers or coaches should pay attention to and design interventions to fix them. For the errors that occasionally appear in beginning students' or athletes' performance, teachers or coaches need to allow time for them to establish consistent performance through more practices.

Beginning students or athletes will also get tired more quickly than those who are experienced and advanced. When determining the number of performance trials for beginning students or athletes, teachers or coaches need to strike a balance. More trials will help teachers or coaches to identify the consistent pattern of beginning students' or athletes' skill performance. However, more performance trials can lead to unintended consequences. Beginning students or athletes will get tired after many performance trials. As a result of fatigue, they will make unnecessary errors. Therefore, when an error occurs, especially after many performance trials, poor physical conditioning may be the cause of this error. Teachers or coaches need to be aware of this situation and make a note during their observation. This information is critical to conducting accurate evaluation and diagnosis and designing appropriate interventions to fix the error.

Nature of the skill

Skills vary in terms of complexity. Some sports skills in nature are more complex and difficult than other sports skills. Observing more complex skills can be more demanding than observing skills that contain much fewer movements. More trials of observations may be needed for complex skills such as triple jump, hammer throwing, and kicking a soccer ball than simple skills such as running, pistol shooting, and archery. For example, gymnastics vault skills involves long distance, high speed, and considerable height and contains complex movements, including a long and fast approach, a takeoff, flight onto and off the horse, and landing. For archery, it consists of eye-on target, pull back string, and release. Given that gymnastics vaulting is more complex and demanding than archery, more trials of observations are necessary for teachers or coaches to gather sufficient data on their students' or athletes' performance for reliable evaluation and diagnosis. When compared to continuous and repetitive skills such as running, discrete sports skills such as golf swing may also require more trials of observations.

Vantage points

A vantage point is an optimal location and angle where teachers or coaches must determine to observe their students' or athletes' performance (Knudson & Morrison, 2002). Appropriate vantage points are critical to successfully gather data during observation. In most cases, the best vantage point for observing a skill is at right angles to the plane of movement at distances of 10 to 15 meters for movements with limited ground speed or being performed in small areas and 20 to 40 meters for fast movements or movements covering a large distance or tall heights (Knudson & Morrison, 2002). The selection of vantage points is often dependent on how complex movements are, how long and high movements cover, and how body movements change over the course of the actions. Therefore, multiple vantage points are needed for movements that are complex, cover long distance, are performed at tall heights, or change from one cardinal plane to another cardinal plane.

Number of observations

Teachers or coaches need to determine how many observations they need to gather sufficient information about their students' or athletes' performance for later evaluation and diagnosis. In general, multiple observations are needed for teachers or coaches to identify a consistent pattern in students' or athletes' performance, thus providing a reliable evaluation and diagnosis of their performance. The recommendations regarding the number of observations varies among researchers. Logan and McKinney (1970) recommended a minimum of eight trials. Hay and Reid (1982) recommended 15 trials as a guideline. Knudson and Morrison (2002) recommended that the number of observations be between five and eight trials for most sports skills. Studies from Morrison and his colleagues (Morrison & Harrison, 1985; Morrison & Reeve, 1989, 1992) showed that five trials are sufficient for consistent qualitive analysis for some sport skills.

We recommend that the number of observations be between five and eight trials. Five-to-eight trial is just a reasonable rule of thumb. Some teachers or coaches may need four or fewer trials for certain sports. Other teachers or coaches may need more than eight trials. Teachers or coaches should have a flexible mindset since there are three major factors affecting how many observations are necessary for information gathering. The nature of skills and characteristics of students or athletes are the first two major factors, which have been discussed in detail above. The last major factor is the levels of content knowledge and experience teachers or coaches possess. The more in-depth content knowledge and experiences, the less observations teachers or coaches coach may need to gather all the necessary data on their students' or athletes' performance. Very often, experienced teachers or coaches who are well knowledgeable of the skill can identify the performance errors in their students or athletes much quicker than those with less experience and content knowledge.

A whole-to-specific approach

Generally, teachers or coaches will use a whole-to-specific approach to conduct observations of performers who are beginning or intermediate. The beginning or intermediate players often make numerous performance errors, which can occur in all three different phases and are inconsistent. In one performance trial, students or athletes perform one element incorrectly. However, in the next performance trial, they perform it correctly. This is very typical given that the beginning or intermediate players are still in the process of establishing their performance patterns. Therefore, to observe a beginning or intermediate player's skill performance, teachers or coaches will watch the whole skill several times to get a complete understanding of students' or athletes' performance, and then home in on the skill's phases and key elements where major performance errors occur in a consistent pattern. For students or athletes who are at advanced levels, teachers or coaches will directly focus their observations on specific key performance errors for interventions, which often occur during the execution phase.

Safety

Teachers or coaches must ensure safety when observing their students' or athletes' performance. They do not want to put themselves or their students or athletes in danger. Where to stand as an observer during observation is critical to ensure safety. For example, if students or athletes perform a basketball layup, teachers or coaches must not stand under the basket. If teachers or coaches stand under the basket, students or athletes can run into them during landing since their body still moves forward. The body collision can lead to physical injuries to either students/athletes or teachers/coaches.

Steps for observation

Teachers or coaches generally go through the following three steps to complete observations. First, teachers or coaches need to decide the goal of the skill, what to look at, what observational instrument to use, and where to stand to avoid conditions that distract themselves and their students or athletes. Then teachers or coaches observe the skill five to eight times from several different vantage points. Finally, teachers or coaches record students' or athletes' performance by completing an observational instrument or a skill analysis sheet and making notes and comments about appropriate and inappropriate movement elements during observation.

Summary

This chapter focuses on the second component of the Integrative Biomechanical Model of Qualitative Skill Analysis: Observation. Eight effective strategies for conducting observation and three steps to observe are discussed. Using those effective strategies and following those steps to conduct observations of students' or athletes' skill performance are critical to gathering important data for evaluation and diagnosis and intervention, which will be introduced in the following two chapters.

Questions for reflection

- What is observation?
- What are eight effective observational strategies? Please describe each strategy in detail.
- What are three steps to observe a skill?

References

Hay, J. G., & Reid, J. G. (1982). *The anatomical and mechanical bases of human motion.* Englewood Cliffs, N.J.: Prentice-Hall.

Knudson, D. V., & Morrison, C. S. (2002). *Qualitative analysis of human movement* (2nd ed.). Champaign, IL: Human Kinetics.

Logan, G. A., & McKinney, W. C. (1970). *Kinesiology.* Dubuque, IA: William C. Brown.

Morrison, C. S., & Harrison, J. M. (1985). Movement analysis and the classroom teacher. *CAHPER Journal, 51*(5), 16–19.

Morrison, C. S., & Reeve, J. (1989). Effect of different video tape instructional units on undergraduate physical education majors' qualitative analysis of skill. *Perceptual and Motor Skills, 69,* 111–114.

Morrison, C. S., & Reeve, J. (1992). Perceptual style and instruction in the acquisition of qualitative analysis of movement by majors in elementary education. *Perceptual and Motor Skills, 74,* 579–583.

15   Evaluation and diagnosis

Outcomes

- Understand what evaluation is.
- Understand what diagnosis is.
- Understand different types of movement errors.
- Conduct evaluation and diagnosis of students' or athletes' skill performance by following the suggested steps.

The third component of the Integrated Biomechanical Model of Qualitative Skill Analysis is evaluation and diagnosis. Through observation, teachers or coaches gather a lot of data on their students' or athletes' skill performance. Those data contain a significant amount of information that teachers or coaches must think through carefully to conduct evaluation and diagnosis. Evaluation and diagnosis are very critical in the process of qualitative skill analysis. A good evaluation and diagnosis lay a critical foundation for successful interventions. The component of evaluation and diagnosis has two parts: evaluation and diagnosis (Knudson & Morrison, 2002).

What is evaluation?

Knudson and Morrison (2002) have defined evaluation as "a judgment of quality, to ascertaining the value or amount of something (p. 112)". Evaluation is to compare actual skill performance with the ideal form of performance based on the biomechanical model and then judge actual performance quality by identifying areas of strengths and weakness for improvement.

   By carefully examining the data collected through observations, teachers or coaches compare their students' or athletes' skill performance with the ideal form of performance based on the biomechanical model and then identify what they performed correctly and what errors they made in their performance. A successful evaluation of students' or athletes' skill performance is not only dependent on how in-depth the knowledge of critical elements of the skill teachers or coaches has but also whether they have the ability to differentiate the actual performance from the ideal form.

DOI: 10.4324/9781003331964-19

Table 15.1 Evaluation of soccer in-step passing

Phase	Critical elements	Present? (yes/no)	Notes
Preparation	Feet shoulder width	Yes	
	Face target	Yes	
	Back straight	Yes	
	Arms at side	Yes	
	Knees bent	Yes	
	Eyes on target	Yes	
Execution	Plant non-kicking foot beside ball (6–8 inches away)	No	Was planted behind the ball
	Toes to the direction of the target	No	Pointing to the left of the target
	Shift weight to plant foot	Yes	
	Swing kicking foot slightly back and then forward toward the ball	Yes	
	Square foot to ball	Yes	
	Make contact with the middle of the ball	No	Contacting the right side of the ball
	Arms swing in opposition	Yes	
Follow through	Follow through with kicking leg	Yes	
	Land on kicking foot	Yes	

As shown in Table 15.1, based on the observation data, teachers or coaches can tell that their students or athletes made three major errors while they performed very well in other aspects of soccer in-step passing skill. The three major errors are the following: (1) students or athletes planted their non-kicking foot behind the ball; (2) the non-kicking foot toes point to the left of the target; and (3) students or athletes contacted the right side of the ball. Based on those data, teachers or coaches can proceed further to diagnose their students' or athletes' skill performance, specifically focusing on those performance errors for better performance.

What is diagnosis?

Knudson and Morrison (2002) have defined diagnosis as "critical scrutiny and judgment in differentiating a problem from its symptoms (pp. 118–119)". Diagnosis is to analyze the causes of performance errors and the relationships among those performance errors, and then prioritize those errors for subsequent interventions. Through evaluation, teachers or coaches identify errors in their students' or athletes' skill performance. Next, teachers or coaches must analyze what causes their students' or athletes' performance errors and determine which error(s) will be fixed first based on the relationships among those errors.

Sources causing performance errors

Researchers have proposed different sources that can cause performance errors. For example, Hoffman (1983) identified critical abilities, skills, or psychosocial factors as causes of movement errors. For a skill error, it can also be further classified as technique-, perception-, and decision-related. Philipp and Wilkerson (1990) classified errors into four categories: bio-mechanical, physiological, perceptual, and psychological. By integrating the classifications of Hoffman (1983) and Philipp and Wilkerson (1990), four sources can contribute to movement errors: physical conditioning, technical deficiency, perception, decision-making, and psychosocial factors. Movement errors can be caused by a deficiency in physical conditioning such as strength and power, agility, flexibility, speed, and endurance etc. Technical errors are related to the deficiency in techniques such as no follow-through when throwing a ball. Decision-making errors are mistakes in making tactical decisions or selecting strategies when performing a skill. Perceptual errors are misunderstanding of technical features or misjudgment of environmental cues. Psychosocial errors are associated with psychological, social, motivational, and emotional factors, which negatively impact students' or athletes' skill performance (Knudson & Morrison, 2002).

A performance error can be attributed to one or a combination of all five sources. Teachers or coaches must first accurately identify which source(s) cause the error and then can design appropriate interventions to fix the error. Different errors require different approaches to correct them. For example, for a performance error due to technical deficiency, teachers or coaches must develop interventions to focus on technical elements of the skill. If students or athletes made a performance error due to lacking arm strength in their golf swing, then teachers or coaches will need to develop a resistance training program to build up their arm strength.

For technical errors, the next step is to understand why and how those errors affect performance using bio-mechanical principles. For example, when performing soccer in-step passing, students or athletes at the beginning level often fail to keep their feet shoulder-width apart and align their toes to target. Three major bio-mechanical principles can be applied to explain how those technical errors affect students' or athletes' performance: balance, stability, and trajectory. Specifically, when students or athletes have a narrow stance, their center of gravity is high. As a result, students or athletes will have poor balance and stability, which will negatively affect the power they will produce. A narrow stance will affect the height at which it is released and the velocity at the moment of release. Thus, it will change the trajectory of the object. More information is provided in Table 15.2. When teachers or coaches can accurately apply bio-mechanical principles to clearly understand why and how those technical errors affect performance, they can design appropriate and effective interventions to fix those errors, thus improving their students' or athletes' performance.

Table 15.2 Application of biomechanical principles in skill analysis of soccer in-step passing

Errors	Underlying biomechanical principles
1 Plant foot not beside the ball	Force/momentum: When you plant your non-kicking foot behind, your center of gravity is far behind the ball. When you swing your kicking foot forward, you contact the ball almost at the end of the range of your leg-kicking motion. This will produce less force/momentum.
2. Toes not pointing to target	Momentum: When toes are not pointing to the target, it will potentially limit the range of motion due to toes pointing to inside. Thus, less power or momentum will be produced.
	Trajectory/direction of force: Trajectory is the combination of horizontal and vertical forces. The trajectory of an object will be affected by a combination of three factors: Angle of release (trajectory angle), velocity at the moment of release, and the height at which it is released. Since the toes are not pointing to the target, the angle and velocity at the moment of release will be impacted. This will affect the trajectory.
3. Kicking foot not square to ball	Trajectory: Since the kicking foot is not square to the ball, it will change the contact points of the foot and the ball. This will change the angle, thus affecting the trajectory of the ball.

Prioritizing performance errors for intervention

The final step in diagnosis is to understand how performance errors relate to one another and prioritize them for interventions. Typically, teachers or coaches must first fix the psychosocial, perceptual, and decision-making errors and then fix the technical errors. One main reason is that those errors can cause the occurrence of technical errors. For technical errors, we generally recommend fixing those in the preparation phase first, and then move on to fix those in the execution and follow-through phases. An execution of a skill is a result of a series of sequential movements of body parts. Body movements in the preparation phase affect those in the execution and follow-through phases. Within the same phase, if one movement error may lead to the other error, we fix the first one first. For example, when throwing a football, two potential technical errors that students or athletes can make are small stepping to target and limited trunk rotation. Limited trunk rotation may be caused by small stepping. Very often, after fixing the stepping error, the trunk rotation issue will also be fixed automatically. Therefore, understanding the relationships among technical errors will help teachers or coaches prioritize which error to fix first, thus improving the effectiveness and efficiency of their teaching or coaching.

Summary

This chapter introduces the third component of the Integrated Biomechanical Model of Qualitative Skill Analysis: evaluation and diagnosis. Evaluation is to compare actual skill performance with the ideal form of performance based on the biomechanical model and then judge actual performance quality by identifying areas of strengths and weakness for improvement. Diagnosis is to analyze the causes of performance errors and the relationships among those performance errors, and then prioritize those errors for subsequent interventions. Evaluation and diagnosis are key in the process of qualitative skill analysis. Accurate evaluation and diagnosis lay a critical foundation for successful interventions. When teachers or coaches can accurately apply biomechanical principles to clearly understand why and how those technical errors affect performance, they can design appropriate and effective interventions to fix those errors, thus improving their students' or athletes' performance. A clear understanding of the relationships among technical errors will help teachers or coaches prioritize which error to fix first, thus improving the effectiveness and efficiency of their teaching or coaching.

Questions for reflection

- What is evaluation?
- What is diagnosis?
- What are different types of performance errors?
- How to successfully conduct evaluation and diagnosis of students' or athletes' skill performance?

References

Hoffman, S. J. (1983). Clinical diagnosis as a pedagogical skill. In T. J. Templin & J. K. Olson (Eds.), *Teaching in physical education* (pp. 35–45). Champaign, IL: Human Kinetics.

Knudson, D. V., & Morrison, C. S. (2002). *Qualitative analysis of human movement* (2nd ed.). Human Kinetics.

Philipp, J. A., & Wilkerson, J. W. (1990). *Teaching team sports: A co-educational approach*. Human Kinetics.

16   Intervention

Outcomes

- Comprehend the definition of intervention.
- Understand the definition of various forms of intervention.
- Use various forms to design effective interventions to maximize students' or athletes' skill performances.

Definition of intervention

Once teachers or coaches evaluate and diagnose their students' or athletes' skill performance based on systematic observation, they will develop interventions to maximize their skill performances. Intervention is the process of actions taken by teachers or coaches to maximize students' or athletes' skill performance (Knudson & Morrison, 2002). The purposes of intervention can be twofold. The first one is to reinforce what students or athletes are performing correctly, which is to provide motivation for continuous practice. The second purpose is to correct skill performance errors among students or athletes, thus making performances better (Knudson & Morrison, 2002). Developmentally appropriate interventions are critical in the process of qualitative skill analysis. Developmentally inappropriate interventions can lead to worse performances among students or athletes, even potential physical injuries, or psychological damage.

Various forms of interventions

There are various forms of interventions that teachers or coaches can use to maximize students' or athletes' performance, including feedback, visual modeling, physical and mechanical assistance, conditioning, psycho-social and emotional intervention, and practices. Which form of intervention to choose depends on the types of errors that students or athletes make in their performance and what cause(s) those errors. In the following sections, various forms of interventions will be discussed with some specific examples.

Feedback

The first most frequently used intervention is to provide feedback to students or athletes on their performance. In Chapter 3 of preparation, we discuss the

DOI: 10.4324/9781003331964-20

definition and various types of feedback. The literature on feedback is also reviewed. Teachers or coaches can provide feedback by using cues or phrases. In some cases, where students or athletes completely fail to understand the skill, teachers or coaches may need to reteach it by providing full instruction again.

Teachers or coaches may also need to use exaggeration or compensation to change their students' or athletes' performance (Knudson & Morrison, 2002). Knudson and Morrison (2002) used tennis serve and basketball shooting as examples to demonstrate how exaggerations or compensation can be used to correct movement errors. For example, beginning students or athletes often shoot a basketball at the rim because of low trajectory at the release point. Teachers or coaches can ask students or athletes to shoot with a higher trajectory by saying "shooting to the sky". When using exaggeration or compensation, teachers or coaches need to be cautious since it can lead to the development of ineffective and inefficient movement patterns. It is recommended that this stimulus should be taken out as soon as students or athletes get the idea of what teachers or coaches intend to communicate to them.

In general, teachers or coaches need to avoid providing general and/or negative feedback to students or athletes. Feedback must be positive, specific, timely, and frequent, which is aligned with students' or athletes' performance. Feedback shall be provided to students or athletes immediately following their practice and as many times as needed. To increase students' or athletes' motivation during practice, teachers or coaches can provide positive and general feedback such as "nice job" or "thumbs up". To remediate students' or athletes' performance errors, teachers or coaches must provide positive and specific feedback, which focuses on the errors made by their students or athletes.

Visual modeling

The second most frequently used intervention is to provide visual modeling. When students or athletes learn a skill for the first time and fail to perform successfully after a couple practice trials, teachers or coaches can re-demonstrate the full skill or key elements of the skill through physical demonstrations, videos, charts, and diagrams. According to social cognitive theories (Bandura, 1986, 1997), observational learning is an important venue for an individual to learn a skill. By using videos, diagrams, charts, and physical demonstrations, students or athletes can form an image of the correct model of performance in their brain, which can provide guidance on what performance to achieve during their practices. Many students or athletes are visual learners. By watching the demonstration again, students or athletes can quickly grasp the essentials of the skill. With the advancement of technology, teachers or coaches can use professional athletes' practice or competition videos from the internet for visual modeling during their teaching or coaching.

Physical and mechanical assistance

In some situations, teachers or coaches provide physical and mechanical assistance to help their students or athletes successfully perform a skill through a physical force or some aids or mechanical devices (Lockhart, 1966) or feel a specific body position or action by holding the body part (Knudson & Morrison, 2002). Physical and mechanical assistance is a common tool that teachers or coaches use in their teaching or coaching. For example, when athletes have difficulty in completing the last repetition of bench press or what is known as "forced reps", coaches or spotters can give the amount of help needed to complete the lift. When athletes perform a backward roll, coaches may give a lift during the rolling backward position to help them complete the skill. Coaches may also use an incline wedge for additional mechanical assistance to help athletes master the backward roll. In physical education, teachers may hold students' throwing elbow in an "L" position when learning to throw a football for them to feel the "L" arm position.

As pointed out by Knudson and Morrison (2002), there are two potential issues related to physical and mechanical assistance. The first one is transferring the new feeling into body movements during practices and unlearning the older or faulty motor programs due to muscle memory. It would be very difficult to unlearn a motor program after the brain creates a long-term muscle memory of the skill with physical and mechanical assistance. Therefore, teachers or coaches should be conscious of the timing of when to withdraw physical and mechanical assistance. Physical and mechanical assistance should be withdrawn as soon as students or athletes get a feeling of body positions or movements. The second problem is that physical and mechanical assistance can increase the risk of injury. For example, during the backward roll motion, if teachers or coaches give a lift too much, it can throw students or athletes off balance and hit their head against the floor.

Conditioning

If students' or athletes' performance errors are due to weakness in physical conditioning such as arm strength, endurance, flexibility etc., then teachers or coaches must first design practices to improve their conditioning rather than to fix their deficiency in skills. For example, when performing a golf swing, students or athletes have perfect technical form with excellent hip and shoulder turn but cannot achieve longer distance due to weak muscle strength. In this instance, teachers or coaches should have students or athletes do resistance training to improve muscle strength involved in golf swing action. Deficiency in physical conditioning can limit students' or athletes' performance. Sometimes, it can cause injuries. Therefore, it is very critical for teachers or coaches to differentiate whether performance errors are due to deficiency in physical conditioning or deficiency in movements.

Psycho-social and emotional interventions

Sometimes, students or athletes are not motivated, have bad attitudes toward practices, or have no confidence when coming to physical education classes or practices. When this happens, you probably can imagine how well students or athletes will perform a skill during practices. They will make numerous errors in performance. For some of those performance errors, students or athletes may have never made in their previous performances. In this scenario, teachers or coaches should realize that psycho-social factors contribute to those performance errors. Rather than continuing to fix performance errors through practices, teachers or coaches should employ strategies to boost their students' or athletes' mentality. First, teachers or coaches need to have a chat with their students or athletes to find out the reasons why they are not motivated, express bad attitudes, or have no confidence. Then, teachers or coaches can use theory-based effective strategies to address their students' or athletes' psycho-social and emotional issues.

Numerous social cognitive theories have been proposed to investigate students' or athletes' motivation and cognition, including goal setting (Locke & Latham, 2013, 2015), achievement goals (Dweck, 1986, 2000; Elliot, 1997, 1999; Nicholls, 1984, 1989), conceptions of ability (Nicholls, 1984, 1989) or implicit theories of ability (Dweck, 2000), self-efficacy (Bandura, 1986, 1997), theory of planned behavior (Ajzen, 1985), self-determination (Deci & Ryan, 2012), interest (Hidi & Harackiewicz, 2000; Hidi & Renninger, 2006), attitudes (Ajzen & Fishbein, 1980), and expectancy and values (Eccles et al., 1983). A complete understanding of those theories and associated research literature will equip teachers or coaches with effective strategies to address students' or athletes' psycho-social and emotional issues that occur in teaching or coaching. For example, teachers or coaches can emphasize the efficacy of effort and mastery of learning and personal improvement to maximize students' or athletes' motivation and use novel practices to stimulate students' or athletes' interest.

Practices

When performance errors are due to deficiency in students' or athletes' technical movements, teachers or coaches sometimes must develop practices to fix the errors, especially when providing feedback, visual modeling, and physical assistance still cannot fix the errors. This form of intervention happens very often during teaching or coaching. For example, when performing blocking in football, athletes very often have a stationary stance upon contact. Running feet is critical for successful blocking since it will create momentum to move the opponent. If athletes don't run their feet on contact, they create less power and momentum, which will make it difficult to brace off the opponent. To fix this error, coaches can have athletes practice a drill of pushing a blocking sled. A sled at practice resembles a person and athletes push it by moving their feet to generate more power and momentum.

Another drill that coaches can do is to have athletes put both hands on the wall with arms locked out, stand back from the wall with a forward lean into the wall, and perform knee drives. Driving legs up with knees bending at 90 degree by pushing both feet against the ground will create more power and momentum.

In Chapter 8, detailed information is provided on how to design task progressions. All the information can be used to guide the development of practices or drills for interventions to fix students' or athletes' performance errors. When developing practices for interventions, teachers or coaches must make sure that those practices are practical and safe for their students or athletes to perform. Sometimes, practice may be a great idea, however, it is not practical and can potentially cause an injury to students or athletes.

Summary

Intervention is the last task of qualitative skill analysis. Developmentally and bio-mechanically sound interventions are critical to fixing students' or athletes' performance errors. Various forms of interventions are available for teachers or coaches to use. Teachers or coaches must select appropriate forms of interventions with a great understanding of underlying bio-mechanical principles based on the sources of students' or athletes' errors.

Questions for reflection

- What is intervention?
- What are various forms of interventions?
- If a third-grade student in physical education uses his or her toes to kick while passing the soccer ball to his or her partner during practice, what are the forms of intervention that a teacher can use to correct this error?

References

Ajzen, I. (1985). From intentions to actions: A theory of planned behavior. In J. Kuhl & J. Beckmann (Eds.), *Action control: From cognition to behavior* (pp. 11–39). Berlin, Heidelber, New York: Springer-Verlag.

Ajzen, I., & Fishbein, M. (1980). *Understanding attitudes and predicting social behavior*. Englewood Cliffs, NJ: Prentice-Hall.

Bandura. A. (1986). *Social foundations of thought and action: A social cognitive theory*. England Cliffs, NJ: Prentice Hall.

Bandura, A. (1997). *Cambridge handbook of psychology, health, and medicine*. Cambridge, Angleterre: Cambridge University Press.

Deci, E. L., & Ryan, R. M. (2012). Motivation, personality, and development within embedded social contexts: An overview of self-determination theory. In R. M. Ryan (Ed.), *Oxford handbook of human motivation* (pp. 85–107). Oxford, UK: Oxford University Press.

Dweck, C. S. (1986). Motivational processes affecting learning. *American Psychologist*, *41*, 1040–1048.

Dweck, C. S. (2000). *Self-theories: Their role in motivation, personality, and development*. New York, NY: Psychology Press.

Eccles, J. S., Adler, T. F., Futterman, R., et al. (1983). Expectancies, values, and academic behaviors. In J. T. Spence (Ed.), *Achievement and achievement motivation* (pp. 75–146). San Francisco, CA: W. H. Freeman.

Elliot, A. J. (1997). Integrating the "classic" and "contemporary" approaches to achievement motivation: A hierarchical model of approach and avoidance achievement motivation. In M. L. Maehr & P. R. Pintrich (Eds.), *Advances in motivation and achievement* (Vol. 10, pp. 143–179). Greenwich, CT: JAI Press.

Elliot, A. J. (1999). Approach and avoidance motivation and achievement goals. *Educational Psychologist, 34*, 169–189.

Hidi, S., & Harackiewicz, J. M. (2000). Motivating the academically unmotivated: A critical issue for the 21st century. *Review of Educational Research, 79*, 151–179.

Hidi, S., & Renninger, K. A. (2006). The four-phase model of interest development. *Educational Psychologist, 41*, 111–127.

Knudson, D. V., & Morrison, C. S. (2002). *Qualitative analysis of human movement* (2nd ed.). Champaign, IL: Human Kinetics.

Locke, E. A., & Latham, G. P. (2013). *New developments in goal setting and task performance*. New York, NY: Routledge.

Locke, E. A., & Latham, G. P. (2015). Breaking the rules: A historical overview of goal-setting theory. In A. J. Elliot (Ed.), *Advances in motivation science* (Vol. 2, pp. 99–126). Oxford, England: Elsevier.

Lockhart, A. (1966). Communicating with the learner. *Quest, 6*, 57–67.

Nicholls, J. G. (1984). Conceptions of ability and achievement motivation. In R. Ames & C. Ames (Eds.), *Research on motivation in education: Student motivation* (pp. 39–73). New York, NY: Academic Press.

Nicholls, J. G. (1989). *The competitive ethos and democratic education*. Cambridge, MA: Harvard University Press.

Index

Note: *Italicized* and **bold** page numbers refer to figure and tables.

For Product Safety Concerns and Information please contact our
EU representative GPSR@taylorandfrancis.com Taylor & Francis
Verlag GmbH, Kaufingerstraße 24, 80331 München, Germany